The Washington Manual™ Outpatient Medicine Survival Guide

D0368274

The Washington Manual™ Outpatient Medicine Survival Guide

Faculty Advisor

Daniel M. Goodenberger, M.D.
Professor of Medicine
Chief, Division of Medical Education
Washington University School of Medicine
Director, Internal Medicine Residency Program
Barnes-Jewish Hospital
St. Louis, Missouri

Contents

Contributing Authors

Audreesh Banerjee, M.D.
Senior Resident
Department of Internal Medicine
Washington University School of
    Medicine
Barnes-Jewish Hospital
St. Louis, Missouri

Eric F. Buch, M.D.
Instructor of Medicine
Department of Internal Medicine
Washington University School of
    Medicine
St. Louis, Missouri

Imran Chishti, M.D.
Attending Psychiatrist
Long-Term Psychiatric Care
St. Louis, Missouri

Jill E. Elwing, M.D.
Fellow, Division of
    Gastroenterology
Department of Internal
    Medicine
Washington University School of
    Medicine
Barnes-Jewish Hospital
St. Louis, Missouri

Helen Y. Kim-James, M.D.
Resident Physician
Department of Dermatology
Washington University School of
    Medicine
Barnes-Jewish Hospital
St. Louis, Missouri

**Robin Ann Kundra, M.D.,
    Ph.D.**
Instructor of Medicine
    and Hospitalist
Department of Internal Medicine
Washington University School of
    Medicine
Barnes-Jewish Hospital
St. Louis, Missouri

Grace A. Lin, M.D.
Chief Resident
Department of Internal Medicine
Washington University School of
    Medicine
Barnes-Jewish Hospital
St. Louis, Missouri

Kevin J. Makati, M.D.
Senior Resident
Department of Internal Medicine
Washington University School of
    Medicine
Barnes-Jewish Hospital
St. Louis, Missouri

Christy Mitchell, M.D.
Senior Resident
Department of Internal
    Medicine
Washington University School of
    Medicine
Barnes-Jewish Hospital
St. Louis, Missouri

Jeanie Park, M.D.
Senior Resident
Department of Internal Medicine
Washington University School of
    Medicine
Barnes Jewish Hospital
St. Louis, Missouri

Georges Saab, M.D.
Fellow, Division of Nephrology
Department of Internal
    Medicine
Washington University School of
    Medicine
Barnes-Jewish Hospital
St. Louis, Missouri

Gregory S. Sayuk, M.D.
Fellow, Division of
    Gastroenterology
Department of Internal Medicine
Washington University School of
    Medicine

CONTRIBUTING AUTHORS

Barnes-Jewish Hospital
Former Chief Resident, Veterans
  Affairs Hospital
St. Louis, Missouri

Jay R. Silverstein, M.D.
Senior Resident
Department of Internal
  Medicine
Washington University School of
  Medicine

Barnes-Jewish Hospital
St. Louis, Missouri

Jason D. Wright, M.D.
Fellow, Department of Obstetrics
  and Gynecology
Division of Gynecologic
  Oncology
Washington University School of
  Medicine
St. Louis, Missouri

Chairman's Note

Medical knowledge is increasing at an exponential rate, and physicians are being bombarded with new facts at a pace that many find overwhelming. The Washington Manual™ Survival Guides were developed in this context for interns, residents, medical students, and other practitioners in need of readily accessible practical clinical information. They therefore meet an important need in an era of information overload.

I would like to acknowledge the authors who have contributed to these books. In particular, Tammy L. Lin, M.D., Series Editor, provided energetic and inspired leadership, and Daniel M. Goodenberger, M.D., Series Advisor, Chief of the Division of Medical Education in the Department of Medicine at Washington University, is a continual source of sage advice. The efforts and outstanding skill of the lead authors are evident in the quality of the final product. I am confident that this series will meet its desired goal of providing practical knowledge that can be directly applied to improving patient care.

Kenneth S. Polonsky, M.D.
Adolphus Busch Professor
Chairman, Department of Medicine
Washington University School of Medicine
St. Louis, Missouri

Series Preface

The Washington Manual™ Survival Guides, a multispecialty series, is designed to provide interns, residents, medical students, or anyone on the front lines of clinical care with quick, practical, essential information in an accessible format. It lets you hit the ground running as you learn the basics of practicing clinical medicine, gain more responsibility, and become a valued team member. Although written individually, they all incorporate series features. Each book takes care to give you an insider's view of how to get things done efficiently and effectively, tips on how to "survive" training, and pearls you will want to pass on in the future. It is similar to receiving a great sign-out from your favorite resident. When faced with an unfamiliar situation, we envision getting timely information and guidance from the survival guide (like you would from your resident) to make appropriate decisions at 3:00 p.m. or 3:00 a.m.

One of the most unique and notable features of this new series is that it was truly a joint effort across subspecialties at Washington University. We were fortunate to have significant departmental support, particularly from Kenneth Polonsky, M.D., whose commitment made this series possible. Every survival guide has the credibility of being written by recent interns, residents, or chief residents in that specialty with input from faculty advisors. We were fortunate to have found outstanding lead authors who were not only highly regarded clinicians and teachers, but who also provided significant leadership and collaborated well together. Their incredible enthusiasm and desire to pass on their hard-earned knowledge, experiences, and wisdom clearly shine through in the series.

Anyone who has been through training will tell you the hours are long, the work is hard, and your energy is limited. With either a print or electronic version of a survival guide by your side, we hope you will work more efficiently, make decisions with more confidence, stay out of trouble, and get that ever-elusive good night's rest.

Tammy L. Lin, M.D., Series Editor
Daniel M. Goodenberger, M.D., Series Advisor

Preface

This book is written as a quick, pocket-sized reference for commonly encountered situations in the outpatient clinic setting. It has been written and edited by Washington University residents and interns for their fellow colleagues on the front lines of patient care. It is not meant to be an all-encompassing synopsis of ambulatory medicine; rather, it covers the most common diseases and situations encountered in an outpatient clinic. It is written assuming that textbooks and Internet resources are available and that attending physicians are nearby for consultation. As our understanding and appreciation of clinical medicine grow, we envision that this book, too, will evolve, and we welcome any comments you may have in improving this reference for future generations of house officers.

The editors would like to acknowlege faculty advisor Dan Goodenberger.

G.A.L.
J.E.E.
G.S.S.

Key to Abbreviations

ABI	ankle/brachial index
DHEA-S	dehydroepiandrosterone sulfate
EGD	esophagogastroduodenoscopy
FDA	U.S. Food and Drug Administration
GBM	glomerular basement membrane
GERD	gastroesophageal reflux disease
GnRH	gonadotropin-releasing hormone
G6PD	glucose-6-phosphate dehydrogenase
HBV	hepatitis B virus
HMG-CoA	hydroxymethylglutaryl coenzyme A
LFTs	liver function tests
MCH	mean corpuscular hemoglobin
MCV	mean corpuscular volume
MEN	multiple endocrine neoplasia
MI	myocardial infarction
MS	multiple sclerosis
NSAIDs	nonsteroidal antiinflammatory drugs
PUVA	pulsed ultraviolet actinotherapy
RDW	RBC distribution width
RV	residual volume
Td	tetanus-diphtheria
TLC	total lung capacity
TPN	total parenteral nutrition
UGI	upper gastrointestinal tract
URI	upper respiratory infection

1 Keys to Survival

It's a jungle out there . . .

- Don't panic.

- Wear comfortable shoes.

- Listen to your patients. They usually will tell you what you need to know.

- Be nice to the nurses. They can help keep your clinic moving and your patients happy.

- Update your patient database after each clinic; you'll appreciate it later.

- Be compulsive. Follow up on labs and tests.

- Be compassionate. A caring word or gesture can go a long way in making your patients feel better.

- Ask for help. You are **not** expected to know everything.

- Eat when you can.

- Sleep when you can.

Approach to the Outpatient Setting

Or, how to succeed in clinic without really trying . . .

The goals of an outpatient visit are to (1) evaluate and treat acute problems, (2) manage chronic disease processes, and (3) maintain and promote health.

- **To do at every visit:** (1) Check vital signs, including blood sugar if the patient is diabetic; (2) obtain a list of current medications (have the patient bring the bottles or a list); and (3) chart review for any recent test results or referrals.

- **Remember: You don't need to address all issues in one visit,** since you expect the patient to return for a follow-up visit.

- **Above all, be your patient's advocate.**

DIFFICULT PATIENT SITUATIONS
See Table 2-1.

PROVIDING CULTURALLY COMPETENT CARE
- When caring for a non–English-speaking patient, have a trained medical interpreter/translator in the room if available. Schedule extra time if possible. Direct your interactions (eye contact, speech) to the patient, not the translator.

- Assess the patient's understanding and conception of what is happening to him or her.

- Evaluate the patient's support system and need for further social services.

- Provide written instructions that can be translated.

PAPERWORK
Charting

Put a note in the patient's chart, either dictated or written. Be sure to include the patient's complaints, physical exam, medications, latest lab data, and plan.

Referrals

When filling out referral forms, include a succinct patient history, any relevant lab or test data, your reason for referring the patient, and the urgency of the referral. Also include your contact information so the specialist can contact you or send correspondence.

TABLE 2-1.
HANDLING DIFFICULT PATIENTS

Patient type	Suggestions
The "Oh, by the way" patient; patient with multiple complaints	Set firm boundaries. Ask patient to pick 1–2 complaints to address at this visit and make a return appointment.
Manipulative (e.g., drug seeking)	Set firm boundaries. Make written contracts and document in the chart. Notify all health care team members of the contract terms. Firmly enforce contract.
Suicidal	If active suicidal or homicidal ideation present, provide an escort to the ED for psychological evaluation. Document proceedings carefully in chart.
Abusive	Safety first. Always place yourself between the patient and the door. Seek nursing assistance and involve security personnel. Remove yourself from the situation if necessary.
Noncompliant	Identify barriers (e.g., financial, motivational, cognitive) to noncompliance.
	Explain the consequences of noncompliance to patient (e.g., high risk of complications from uncontrolled diabetes or HTN).
	Provide such aids as pillboxes and written instructions, especially for elderly patients.
Hypochondriac	See patient often and provide a listening ear and reassurance.
	Avoid tests and procedures unless absolutely necessary.
Financially constricted	Talk with the social worker about programs for which your patient may be eligible.
	Work with the pharmacist for medication samples or discounts. (Many drug companies have medication assistance programs.)
	Find lower-cost alternatives for prescription medications.
"Medication intolerant"	Explain that all medications have side effects that are part of the treatment. Explain *expected* side effects of medication.
	Treat symptomatic side effects.
	Consider switching medications.

Lab and Radiology Requisitions

Be sure to specify the test you want and, in the case of radiology tests, a brief patient history (one line), your reason for ordering the test, and any special requests.

Forms Your Patient May Ask You to Fill Out

- **Disability forms:** Various forms from employers, insurance companies, Social Security Administration. Will ask you to assess the patient, describe the disability, and estimate the length of disability.

- **Family and Medical Leave Act:** Allows employees to take time off without losing their jobs if they have a qualifying medical condition or if the leave is to care for an ill family member.

- **Handicapped parking permits:** Certifies that a patient has a disability that makes him or her eligible for a handicapped parking permit.

- **Certification of need for medical supplies:** For such materials as diabetic supplies, wheelchairs, and hospital beds.

- **Work excuses:** Use your judgment about what is reasonable. Be sure to put on the note the days the patient missed, when the patient is able to resume work duties, and any restrictions to work duties (e.g., no lifting of objects >10 lbs, desk work only). Make sure it is on hospital or clinic stationery.

- Above all, ***do not lie***: fill out these forms to the best of your ability and put a copy in the chart.

STAFF RELATIONS

- Remember that you are part of a multidisciplinary health care team. Everyone's goal is the same: to provide the patient with the best possible health care.

- Professional and courteous behavior is essential at all times.

- A little respect goes a long way. (So does an occasional compliment.)

- Give feedback in a constructive and nonjudgmental manner.

- If you have a problem with a staff member, talk directly to that person and try to solve your differences of opinion professionally.

- Settle disagreements privately. ***Never*** argue in front of a patient. If a disagreement cannot be settled, involve a third party, such as an attending physician.

COMMUNITY RESOURCES

- **Social workers** are your best source of local resources regarding assistance for which your patients may qualify.

- **Local agencies,** such as the county health department, offer services including STD and HIV testing and treatment, education, and mental health programs.

- **Free or low-cost clinics** are available in most locales for patients without health insurance.

- **State agencies,** such as the Division of Aging, can be helpful in providing chore workers, safety assessments, and lists of licensed adult day care programs.

- **Community and nonprofit groups** with services in most areas:

  - **Local self-help groups:** Alcoholics Anonymous, Narcotics Anonymous, Gambler's Anonymous, and others.

  - **Disease-specific organizations:** Alzheimer's Association, American Cancer Society, American Diabetes Association, American Heart Association, American Lung Association, Crohn's and Colitis Foundation of America, and others.

  - **Hospice:** provides end-of-life care for terminally ill patients.

  - **Meals on Wheels:** provides hot meals to homebound seniors.

  - **National Council on Alcoholism and Drug Abuse:** provides education and resources for alcoholics and patients addicted to drugs.

  - **Salvation Army:** provides shelter, food, and clothing; may also have drug and alcohol treatment programs.

- **Shelters** are available for homeless persons and victims of domestic violence. Encourage any victims of domestic violence to seek safe shelter as soon as possible.

- **Home health care agencies** can provide home nursing care, home physical therapy, and other assistance for those patients in need of home medical care.

- The **Veteran's Administration** provides services, including medical care, to all veterans.

END-OF-LIFE ISSUES

Discuss with your patients who will make decisions for them if they are unable to do so. Options for ensuring their wishes are carried out at the end of life:

- The **durable power of attorney** (DPOA) for health care is a person designated by the patient to make health care decisions in cases in which the patient is not able to do so. If no DPOA has been appointed, the next of kin becomes the surrogate decision maker. *This document is separate from a DPOA for finances; the two are not interchangeable!*

- A **living will** lays out specific directions for specific circumstances (e.g., no intubation or mechanical ventilation, no admission to a nursing home).

- Document **code status** in the chart. Be specific when addressing level of care (e.g., do not resuscitate/do not intubate, no CPR, no pressors, no antibiotics, no blood transfusions).

Consider recommending nursing home placement, extended care, or an assisted living facility if the patient no longer can safely live at home. Hospice is an option for terminally ill patients who wish to remain at home.

Tools of the Trade

3

There's no room for loose screws . . .

REFERENCES TO CARRY

- Lin T, Rypkema S, eds. *The Washington manual of ambulatory therapeutics*. Philadelphia: Lippincott Williams & Wilkins, 2002.
- *Tarascon pocket pharmacopoeia*. Loma Linda, CA: Tarascon Publishing, 2001.
- Gilbert DN, Moellering RC, Sande MA, eds. *The Sanford guide to antimicrobial therapy*. Hyde Park, VT: Antimicrobial Therapy Inc, 2001.

INSTRUMENTS FOR YOUR POCKET

- Stethoscope
- Reflex hammer
- Microfilament
- Penlight

FOR YOUR PDA
Drug References

- **ePocrates:** Drug database that lists dosages, contraindications, adverse reactions, drug interactions, and approximate cost for each drug; www.epocrates.com
- **ePocrates qID:** Lists recommended therapies for specific infections; hyperlinked with ePocrates; www.epocrates.com
- **ePharmacopoeia:** PDA version of the pocket drug book; www.tarasconpublishing.com/store/palm.asp

Calculations

- **MedCalc:** Database of commonly used formulas; just plug in the numbers. www.netxperience.org/medcalc/index2.html
- **MedMath:** Another database of common formulas; www.mail.med.upenn.edu/~pcheng/medmath/

Databases

- **PatientKeeper:** Database for patient information; www.patientkeeper.com
- **Pocket MD:** www.pocketmd.com

Other Useful Sites

- **AvantGo:** Download websites to your PDA; www.avantgo.com
- **PDA MD:** Contains news reviews, columns, forums, products; www.pdamd.com

INTERNET RESOURCES

General Sites

- www.acponline.org (American College of Physicians)
- www.ama-assn.org (American Medical Association)
- www.healthfinder.org (U.S. Department of Health and Human Services)
- www.mdconsult.com (MD Consult)
- www.medscape.com (Medscape)
- www.guideline.gov (National Guidelines Clearinghouse)
- www.nlm.nih.gov (National Library of Medicine, access to PubMed)
- www.merckmedicus.com (Merck Medicus)

Allergy

- www.aafa.org (Asthma and Allergy Foundation of America)
- www.niaid.nih.gov (National Institute of Allergy and Infectious Diseases)

Cardiology

- www.acc.org (American College of Cardiology)
- www.americanheart.org (American Heart Association)
- www.heartinfo.org (Heart Information Network)
- www.nhlbi.nih.gov (National Heart, Lung, and Blood Institute)

Cerebrovascular Disease

- www.ninds.nih.gov (National Institute of Neurological Diseases)
- www.stroke.org (National Stroke Foundation)

Endocrinology

- www.diabetes.org (American Diabetes Association)
- www.endo-society.org (The Endocrine Society)
- www.niddk.nih.gov (National Institute of Diabetes and Digestive and Kidney Disease)
- www.thyroid.org (American Thyroid Association)

Gastroenterology

- www.acg.gi.org (American College of Gastroenterology)
- www.gastro.org (American Gastroenterological Association)
- www.ccfa.org (Crohn's and Colitis Foundation of America)

Geriatrics

- www.alzheimers.org (Alzheimer's disease)
- www.aoa.dhhs.gov/elderpage.html (Administration on Aging)

Infectious Disease

- www.cdc.gov (Centers for Disease Control and Prevention)
- hivinsite.ucsf.edu (University of California San Francisco's HIV site)
- www.niaid.nih.gov (National Institute of Allergy and Infectious Diseases)
- www.who.int (World Health Organization)

Nephrology

- www.kidney.org (National Kidney Foundation)
- www.niddk.nih.gov (National Institute of Diabetes and Digestive and Kidney Diseases)
- www.renalnet.org (RenalNet)

Oncology

- www.cancer.org (American Cancer Society)
- cancertrials.nci.nih.gov (National Cancer Institute's list of clinical trials)
- www.nci.nih.gov (National Cancer Institute)

Pulmonary

- www.chestnet.org (American College of Chest Physicians)
- www.emphysemafoundation.org (National Emphysema Foundation)

Rheumatology

- www.arthritis.org (The Arthritis Foundation)
- www.nih.gov/niams (National Institute of Arthritis and Musculo-skeletal and Skin Diseases)
- www.rheumatology.org (American College of Rheumatology)

Online Journals

- www.acponline.org/journals/annals/annaltoc.html (*Annals of Internal Medicine*)

- www.aafp.org (*American Family Physician*)

- www.bmj.org (*British Medical Journal*)

- www.jama.ama-assn.org (*JAMA*)

- www.thelancet.com (*The Lancet*)

- www.nejm.org (*New England Journal of Medicine*)

Evidence-Based Medicine Sites

- http://cochranelibarary.net (The Cochrane Database of Systemic Reviews)

- http://www.acponline.org/journals/acpjc/jcmenu.htm (American College of Physicians Journal Club)

4

Telephone Triage

Help, someone call a doctor . . .

INTRODUCTION

Telephone triage is one of the most difficult things to learn during intern year. Calls from your clinic patients happen early and often and range from requests for medication refills to descriptions of chest pain. Your job, based on a short phone conversation, is to decide what course of action should be pursued.

When listening to your patient, ask yourself the following questions:

- What is the complaint? Is it acute, subacute, or chronic?
- What are the patient's underlying medical problems?
- What medications does this patient usually take?
- Can the patient wait until his or her next clinic appointment, or should the issue be addressed sooner?
- Does the patient need to go to the ED? **The most important question is whether the patient should be seen emergently.** The "red flags" listed in Table 4-1 indicate that you should send your patient to the ER.

Once you've decided that your patient does not need to go to the ED, decide whether the patient should be seen before his or her next clinic appointment, or whether the problem can be taken care of without a visit. Use your common sense: When in doubt, arrange for the patient to be seen by a physician in either the clinic or the ED.

COMMON CALLS
Prescription Refills

- Be sure to have the patient leave his or her pharmacy number with you.
- Consider declining refills or giving only one refill of prescriptions if the patient has not been seen in clinic for more than a year, particularly if the patient has multiple medical problems.

Medication Side Effects

All medications have side effects, and patients should be educated about them. Encourage the patient to stick with the medication, as many side effects wane over time. Consider seeing the patient in clinic and changing medications if the side effects are intolerable to the patient.

TABLE 4-1.
RED FLAGS FOR TELEPHONE TRIAGE

Chest pain	Persistent nausea and vomiting
Acute dyspnea	Head trauma
Severe headache	Hip trauma
High fever	Stroke/TIA symptoms
Severe abdominal pain	Syncope
Significant GI bleeding	Altered mental status

Abdominal Pain

Abdominal pain is a tough problem. If the patient has any red flags, have him or her evaluated in the clinic or ED. See Chap. 13, Gastroenterology, for more details and suggested evaluation. If no red flags are present, phone follow-up within a day or two to ensure resolution is reasonable.

Cold and Flu Symptoms

- Most cold and flu symptoms are viral, and patients do not need to be seen.

- Recommend increased rest, fluid intake, and over-the-counter cold remedies for symptomatic treatment. You may offer prescriptions for such drugs as cough medicine and decongestants.

- Remind patients that their symptoms may last for several days. If symptoms persist, follow-up in clinic is necessary.

Cough

- The differential diagnosis of cough is broad; see Chap. 21, Pulmonary Disease.

- Consider over-the-counter or prescription cough medicines (e.g., Robitussin DM, Robitussin AC) for symptomatic relief.

- Remind patients to stop smoking.

- If patient is on an ACE inhibitor, consider having him or her stop it for a few days to see if the cough improves.

Diarrhea

- Most often, diarrhea is due to food poisoning or viral gastroenteritis.

- Generally requires only symptomatic treatment, such as loperamide (Imodium), plus an increased intake of fluids.

- You may need to see the patient if the diarrhea persists, or if there is a significant amount of blood (see Chap. 13, Gastroenterology).

Exacerbations of Chronic Problems

Asthma

- Patients who are in the danger zone (peak flows <50% normal) should be seen in the ED.

- For patients who have persistent symptoms not relieved by short-acting beta-agonists, consider starting a steroid taper and making a follow-up appointment within 1–2 days.

Chronic Obstructive Pulmonary Disease

- Patients who are having a COPD exacerbation likely should be evaluated in an acute care setting (e.g., ED or urgent care).

Congestive Heart Failure

- You may be called with increasing lower extremity edema and/or increasing shortness of breath. Consider increasing the dose of or adding a diuretic, and arrange for the patient to follow up with you within the next week.

Diabetes

- Calls regarding hyper- or hypoglycemia are common. Consider increasing or decreasing insulin doses or PO hypoglycemics as appropriate.

- Ask the patient to keep a blood sugar log, note when the change in dose took place, and then bring the log in to his or her next clinic appointment.

Hypertension

- You may be called about high BP readings. For systolic BP >200 or systolic BP >160 with symptoms (chest pain, shortness of breath, TIA, focal neuro deficits), the patient should be evaluated in the ED. For all others, arrange to see the patient promptly.

Chronic Pain

- Ask about factors that may have exacerbated pain (e.g., recent injury, increased physical activity).

- Consider increasing the dose of or adding a pain medication. Have the patient call you if the new regimen does not give him or her relief.

Falls and Other Injuries

- Always ask about head trauma, symptoms of significant head trauma (severe headache, persistent dizziness, blurred vision, altered mental status), and hip trauma. Such trauma patients should be evaluated in the ED.

- For minor falls and injuries, recommend rest, ice/heat packs, and over-the-counter pain medications. Follow up with the patient within 2 wks.

Urinary Tract Infection

- For patients with symptomatic UTIs, particularly young, healthy women, consider starting therapy empirically with phone follow-up for resolution of symptoms.

- For complicated UTIs, have the patient come into clinic for a urine culture before starting antibiotics. Advise the patient to drink plenty of fluids and seek further medical attention for any red-flag symptoms.

Vaginal Yeast Infections

- Recommend over-the-counter preparations or prescription antifungals.

- If the patient has persistent yeast infections, consider having the patient follow up in clinic for further evaluation (e.g., to check for diabetes).

It's just a little stick . . .

COMPLETE METABOLIC PANEL
Sodium (Na⁺)

- **Elevated in:** Water losses (GI, hyperpnea, sweat), diuresis (diuretic drugs, diabetes mellitus, diabetes insipidus), excess intake (diet, IV fluids), hyperaldosteronism, Cushing's syndrome
- **Decreased in:** Dilutional (congestive heart failure, nephrotic syndrome, cirrhosis, polydipsia, SIADH), Na⁺ loss (vomiting, diarrhea, sweat, diuretics, Addison's disease)

Potassium (K⁺)

- **Elevated in:** Spurious cases (hemolysis, ischemic blood draw), redistribution (extreme exercise, tissue necrosis/trauma, acidosis, aldosterone deficiency, spironolactone, beta blockers, digitalis toxicity), decreased renal clearance (acute renal failure [ARF], chronic renal failure), increased intake (dietary, KCl, IV fluid)
- **Decreased in:** Redistribution (beta-agonists, insulin, alkalosis), inadequate intake, GI losses (diarrhea, laxative abuse, vomiting), renal losses (diuretics, renal tubular acidosis), glucocorticoids, Cushing's syndrome, hyperaldosteronism, licorice

Bicarbonate (HCO_3^-)

- **Elevated in:** Vomiting, gastric suction (H⁺ loss), hyperaldosteronism, metabolic alkalosis, barbiturates, steroids
- **Decreased in:** Metabolic acidosis (renal failure, diabetic ketoacidosis, starvation), salicylate toxicity, diarrhea, thiazide diuretics

Blood Urea Nitrogen (BUN)

- **Elevated in:** Renal disease (chronic renal insufficiency, ARF, urinary tract obstruction), dehydration, GI bleeding, drugs (steroids, lithium, diuretics), high-protein diet
- **Decreased in:** Liver disease, nephrotic syndrome, malnutrition, overhydration, low-protein diet

Creatinine

- **Elevated in:** Renal insufficiency (acute or chronic, renal hypoperfusion), UTI, rhabdomyolysis, diuretics

- **Decreased in:** Low muscle mass (elderly, amputee), debilitation, pregnancy

Calcium (Ca^{2+})

- **Elevated in:** Hyperparathyroidism, malignancy (hematologic, parathyroid hormone related peptide [PTHrP]–producing, bony involvement), excess vitamin D, sarcoidosis, milk-alkali syndrome, hyperthyroidism, thiazide diuretics
- **Decreased in:** Hypoparathyroidism, hypoalbuminemia, chronic renal disease (hyperphosphatemia), osteomalacia, insufficient Ca^{2+} or vitamin D intake, malabsorption

Alanine Aminotransferase (ALT, SGPT)

- **Elevated in:** Liver disease (hepatitis, cirrhosis, hepatic congestion/congestive heart failure, mononucleosis, obstructive jaundice, shock), muscular (MI, myocarditis, muscle trauma/injury, polymyositis), drugs (antibiotics, narcotics, statins, amiodarone, phenytoin), pancreatitis

Aspartate Aminotransferase (AST, SGOT)

- **Elevated in:** Liver disease (hepatitis, cirrhosis, hepatic congestion/congestive heart failure, mononucleosis, obstructive jaundice, shock), muscular (MI, myocarditis, muscle trauma/injury, polymyositis), drugs (antibiotics, narcotics, statins, amiodarone, dilantin), pancreatitis
- **Decreased in:** Renal disease (ARF, hemodialysis), diabetic ketoacidosis

Alkaline Phosphatase

- **Elevated in:** Liver disease (biliary obstruction, cirrhosis, infiltrative, fatty liver), bone disease (Paget's disease, osteomalacia, hypervitaminosis D, fracture, bony metastasis), hyperparathyroidism, hyperthyroidism, drugs (estrogens, antibiotics [erythromycin], phenothiazines), pregnancy
- **Decreased in:** Hypothyroidism, anemia, hypophosphatemia, malnutrition

Albumin

- **Elevated in:** Dehydration
- **Decreased in:** Liver disease, nephrotic syndrome, malnutrition, protein-losing enteropathy, malignancy, chronic inflammatory disease, pregnancy, oral contraceptives

Total Protein

- **Elevated in:** Dehydration, multiple myeloma, Waldenström's macroglobulinemia, sarcoidosis, collagen vascular disease

- **Decreased in:** Malnutrition, low-protein diet, overhydration, malabsorption, pregnancy, malignancy, chronic disease, cirrhosis, nephrotic syndrome

Bilirubin (Direct)

- **Elevated in:** Extrahepatic obstruction (tumor, inflammation, gallstones), drug-induced cholestasis, hereditary disorders (Dubin-Johnson, Rotor's syndrome)

Bilirubin (Indirect)

- **Elevated in:** Hemolysis, liver disease (hepatitis, cirrhosis, malignancy, hepatic congestion), hereditary disorders (Gilbert's disease, Crigler-Najjar syndrome)

DUAL-ENERGY X-RAY ABSORPTIOMETRY (DEXA) SCAN

- **Indication:** Measures hip and spine bone density as markers for osteopenia and subsequent risk for fracture. Indicated for all patients at risk for osteoporosis (see Chap. 10, Endocrinology).

- **Interpretation:**
  - **T score:** Number of standard deviations above or below the mean bone density vs. young controls.
  - **Z score:** Number of standard deviations above or below the mean bone density vs. age-matched controls.

WHO guidelines for diagnosis of osteopenia/osteoporosis (based on T score) are featured in Table 5-1.

FASTING LIPID PANEL

- **Indication:** To measure a patient's lipids, including total cholesterol, low-density lipoprotein cholesterol, high-density lipoprotein (HDL) cholesterol, triglycerides (TGs), as a risk factor for coronary artery disease.

TABLE 5-1.
WHO GUIDELINES FOR OSTEOPOROSIS

T Score	Diagnosis
>−1	Normal
−1 to −2.5	Osteopenia
<−2.5	Osteoporosis
<−2.5 with fracture	Severe osteoporosis

- **Interpretation:**

  - Patient must be fasting ≥8 hrs before test for accurate results, particularly for TGs and low-density lipoprotein (calculated based on total cholesterol, HDL, and TGs).

  - Initial evaluation with total cholesterol and HDL only, or with complete lipid panel.

  - For treatment guidelines, see Chap. 8, Cardiology, Table 8-10.

HEMOGLOBIN A₁c

- **Indication**: Measurement of glycemic control over 3 mos in diabetic patients.

- **Interpretation:**

  - Normal range will vary by lab and method used; generally 4–8%.

  - Useful as a tool to follow chronic blood sugar levels and therapeutic efficacy, particularly in those patients whose sugars fluctuate widely.

  - **Test interval:** Consider ordering q3mos for uncontrolled diabetes or if changing treatment regimen, q6mos if diabetes controlled.

  - See Chap. 10, Endocrinology, for guidelines on treatment.

INR MONITORING

- **Indication:** Monitoring of warfarin therapy (see Table 5-2 for guidelines). Monitor as often as necessary (q1–2wks) until at stable dose, then q4–6wks.

MAMMOGRAPHY

- **Indication:**

  - Screening: For patients with no complaints or abnormalities on exam. All women ≥50 should be screened (recommendations for initiation vary by organization). See Chap. 7, Health Maintenance and Preventive Medicine, for detailed recommendations.

  - Diagnostic: For patients with abnormalities on exam. Involves additional views.

- **Interpretation:**

  - Mammography can detect masses, calcifications, or abnormal areas of breast tissue that may indicate breast disease. Findings are generally graded according to the American College of Radiology BIRAD categories (Table 5-3).

TABLE 5-2.
GUIDELINES FOR INR MONITORING

Indication	Target INR	Duration
Deep venous thrombosis/pulmonary embolism	2.0–3.0	6 mos to lifelong (for recurrent events)
Cerebrovascular accident	2.0–3.0	Lifelong
Atrial fibrillation	2.0–3.0	Lifelong
Mitral valve prolapse + history of atrial fibrillation, recurrent TIA, cerebrovascular accident, mitral regurgitation, congestive heart failure	2.0–3.0	Lifelong
St. Jude's valve in aortic position	2.0–3.0	Lifelong
Mechanical prosthetic valves (except St. Jude's)	2.5–3.5	Lifelong

TABLE 5-3.
AMERICAN COLLEGE OF RADIOLOGY BIRAD CATEGORIES

Category	Definition	Comment
0	Needs additional imaging evaluation	May need extra views and/or U/S.
1	Negative	No masses, calcifications, or architectural disturbances are present.
2	Benign finding	Contains typically benign findings (calcified fibroadenoma); no short-interval follow-up required.
3	Probably benign finding—short-interval follow-up recommended.	Findings show very high probability of being benign; demonstration of stability preferable to immediate biopsy.
4	Suspicious abnormality—biopsy should be considered.	Appearance not characteristic of malignancy; however, probability of malignancy is sufficiently high to include biopsy as consideration.
5	Highly suggestive of malignancy; appropriate action should be taken.	High probability of malignancy; referral to specialist indicated.

D'Oris CJ, Bassett LW, Feig SA, et al. *Illustrated breast imaging reporting and data system*, 3rd ed. Reston, VA: American College of Radiology, 1998.

TABLE 5-4.
BETHESDA SYSTEM OF PAP SMEAR INTERPRETATION

Category	Management
Within normal limits	Routine follow-up.
Benign cellular changes:	
Infection (e.g., *Trichomonas*, *Candida*, *Actinomyces*, herpes simplex virus)	Treat infection; routine follow-up.
Reactive changes (e.g., inflammation, atrophy, IUD)	Likely no need for treatment; routine follow-up.
Atypical squamous cells of undetermined significance (ASCUS)	*Options:* 1. Follow-up Pap q4–6mos for 2 yrs. •If negative for 2 consecutive Paps, resume routine screening interval. • If a smear again shows ASCUS, consider colposcopy. 2. If postmenopausal, treat with estrogen cream for 6 wks, then repeat Pap; if ASCUS persists, consider colposcopy. 3. If high-risk patient in whom follow-up is questionable, consider colposcopy. 4. DNA testing for high-risk types of HPV can be done. If positive, colposcopy is recommended.
Low-grade squamous intraepithelial lesion (encompasses CIN 1, HPV, and mild dysplasia)	*Options:* 1. Colposcopy is recommended for all premenopausal women. 2. For postmenopausal women, treat with estrogen cream for 6 wks, then repeat Pap; if persistently positive, consider colposcopy.
High-grade squamous intraepithelial lesion (encompasses moderate/severe dysplasia, CIN 2,3)	Colposcopy and directed biopsy
Squamous cell carcinoma	Refer to gynecology
Atypical glandular cells of undetermined significance	Refer to gynecology for colposcopy with endocervical or endometrial sampling
Endocervical adenocarcinoma	Refer to gynecology
Endometrial adenocarcinoma	Refer to gynecology

Adapted from Solomon D, Davey D, Kurman R, et al. The 2001 Bethesda System: terminology for reporting results of cervical cytology. *JAMA* 2002;287:2114–2119; and Wright TC, Cox JT, Massad LS. Consensus guidelines for management of women with cervical cytological abnormalities. *JAMA* 2002; 287:2120–2129.

- Younger women are more likely to have false-positive and false-negative results on mammography owing to breast density.

PAP SMEAR

- **Indication:** Detects abnormal cervical cells as screening for cervical cancer. Consider all women who are sexually active or >18 for screening.
- **Interpretation:** See Table 5-4.

PULMONARY FUNCTION TESTS

- **Indication:** Used to assess volumes, function, and diffusing capacity of the lungs; assess severity of such lung diseases as asthma or COPD.
- **Interpretation:**
  - **Lung volumes:** See Fig. 5-1.
  - **FEV_1:** Amount of air expired during the first second of expiration.
    - **FVC:** Forced vital capacity.
    - **Bronchodilator response:** Improvement in FEV_1 or

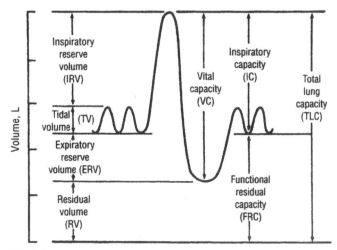

FIG. 5-1.
Lung volume interpretation. TLC = TV + IRV + ERV + RV; IC = TV + IRV; FRC = ERV + RV; VC = TV + IRV + ERV. (From Grippi MA, Metzger LF, et al. Pulmonary function testing. In: Fishman AP, ed., *Pulmonary diseases and disorders*, 2nd ed. New York: McGraw-Hill, 1988, with permission.)

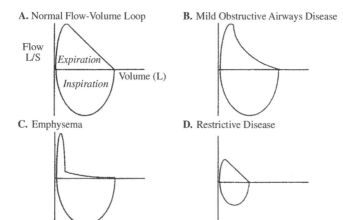

A. Normal Flow-Volume Loop   **B.** Mild Obstructive Airways Disease

C. Emphysema   **D.** Restrictive Disease

FIG. 5-2.
A: Normal flow-volume loop. **B:** Flow-volume loop showing mild obstructive airways disease. **C:** Flow-volume loop showing emphysema. **D:** Flow-volume loop showing restrictive disease. (From Karnik AM, Khan FA. Interpretation of pulmonary function test. *Resid Staff Physician* 1999;45(4):53, with permission.)

FVC of $\geq 12\%$ and >200 cc after beta-agonist administration; useful in detecting asthma and any reversible component of COPD.

- **DLCO/VA:** Diffusion capacity of carbon monoxide across the lungs, corrected for alveolar volume; decreased in anemia, lung resection, lung fibrosis, emphysema (but DLCO/VA is normal in chronic bronchitis).

- **Flow-volume loops:** See Fig. 5-2.

  - **Obstructive flow-volume loops:** Asthma, emphysema.

  - **Restrictive flow-volume loops:** Space-occupying lesions (e.g., pneumonia, pleural effusion, tumor), respiratory muscle weakness (e.g., neuromuscular diseases), interstitial fibrosis, chest wall abnormalities (e.g., kyphoscoliosis, ankylosing spondylitis), hemidiaphragm elevation (e.g., pregnancy, obesity, ascites).

URINALYSIS

- **Indications:** Any patient with urinary symptoms; all pregnant women on a periodic basis.

- **Interpretation:**
  - **Urine dipstick:** Gives primarily qualitative and limited quantitative information about a urine specimen. Usually includes urine pH, specific gravity, protein, glucose, ketones, blood, bilirubin, nitrites, leukocyte esterase.
    - **Proteinuria:** Renal diseases, such as nephrotic syndrome, nephritic syndrome, renal tubular disease, pyelonephritis, polycystic kidney disease; also in pregnancy, multiple myeloma, acute illnesses.
    - **Glucosuria:** Diabetes, Cushing's syndrome, hemachromatosis, pancreatitis, CNS disorders, renal tubular dysfunction, pregnancy; also can be caused by such medications as thiazide diuretics, corticosteroids, and oral contraceptives.
    - **Ketonuria:** Uncontrolled diabetes (diabetic ketoacidosis), starvation, alcoholics.
    - **Blood:** Hemolytic anemias, glomerulonephritis, nephrolithiasis, UTI, polycystic kidney disease, trauma, tumor, acute tubular necrosis, renal infarction, myoglobin.
    - **Bilirubinuria:** Liver disease, obstruction of biliary tract, congenital hyperbilirubinemias.
    - **Leukocyte esterase:** Indicative of pyuria, infection.
    - **Nitrite:** Indicative of infection. May be negative in infection, as some bacteria do not reduce nitrate to nitrite.
  - **Microscopic exam:** Usually includes RBC count, WBC count, bacteria count, number of casts.
    - **RBCs:** If dipstick (+) for blood but no RBCs on microscopy, consider myoglobinuria.
    - **WBCs:** If WBCs present, confirms infection.
    - **Casts:** Hyaline (normal), RBC cast (abnormal), WBC cast (abnormal), granular (abnormal).

SUGGESTED READING

Bakerman S. *Bakerman's ABC's of interpretive laboratory data*, 3rd ed. Myrtle Beach, SC: Interpretive Laboratory Data, 1994.

Karnik AM, Khan FA. Interpretation of pulmonary function tests: a step-by-step algorithmic approach. *Resid Staff Physician* 1999; 45(4):45–63.

White TC, Cox JT, Massad LS. 2001 Consensus guidelines for management of women with cervical cytological abnormalities. *JAMA* 2002;287:2120–2129.

Useful Formulae

Anyone have a calculator?

ANION GAP (AG)

- AG = $[Na^+] - ([Cl^-] + [HCO_3^-])$
- Normal: 8–12 mEq/L

BODY MASS INDEX (BMI)

- BMI = weight (kg)/height (m^2) or weight (lbs)/height ($in.^2$) × 704.5
- <18.5 = underweight
- 18.5–24.9 = normal weight
- 25–29.9 = overweight
- >30 = obese

IDEAL BODY WEIGHT (IBW)

- For men: 50 kg + 2.3 kg/in. for every in. >60" (5 ft)
- For women: 45.5 kg + 2.3 kg/in. for every in. >60" (5 ft)
- >20% over IBW considered obese

CORRECTED SERUM CALCIUM

- Corrected $[Ca^{2+}]$ = [(4.0 – serum albumin) × 0.8] + serum $[Ca^{2+}]$

CREATININE CLEARANCE (CrCl)

- Measured (24-hr urine): CrCl = U_{cr} × urine volume/P_{Cr} × time.
- Calculated: [(140 – age) × weight (kg)/S_{cr} × 72] × 0.85 for female.
- Normal: >100 mL/min.
- Adjust medication dosages if CrCl <50.

MICROALBUMIN:CREATININE RATIO (M:C RATIO)

- M:C ratio = urine albumin (mg/L)/ urine Cr (mg/dL) × 100.
- <30 = normal.
- 30–300 = microalbuminuria.
- >300 = macroalbuminuria.
- Urine dipstick tests for protein are not sensitive for the detection of microalbuminuria, as a positive test indicates gross proteinuria.

CORRECTED RETICULOCYTE COUNT

- Corrected reticulocyte count = reticulocyte count × (Hct/45%).

- Correction factor for patient's anemia, as degree of reticulocytosis is dependent on patient's Hct.

- Normal <2 (for patients with normal hematocrit).

- For anemic patients, good marrow response = 2.0–6.0.

MEDICAL EPIDEMIOLOGY

Test result	Disease (+)	Disease (−)
Test (+)	True positive (A)	False positive (B)
Test (−)	False negative (C)	True negative (D)

Sensitivity = A/(A + C)

- Measures the number of patients with a disease who have a positive test result.

- The higher the sensitivity of a test, the more likely it is to detect patients with the disease.

Specificity = B/(B + D)

- Measures the number of patients without a disease who have a negative test result.

- The more specific a test, the more likely it is to rule out patients without the target disorder.

Positive predictive value (PPV) = A/(A + B)

- The percentage of patients with a positive test result in whom the disease is present.

- PPV also depends on the *prevalence* of a disorder in the population.

Negative predictive value (NPV) = D/(C + D)

- The percentage of patients with a negative test result in whom the disease is absent.

- NPV depends on the *prevalence* of the disease in the population as well.

Prevalence

The number of patients in a given population who have the disease at one time (e.g., the number of Americans who currently have the diagnosis of type II diabetes mellitus).

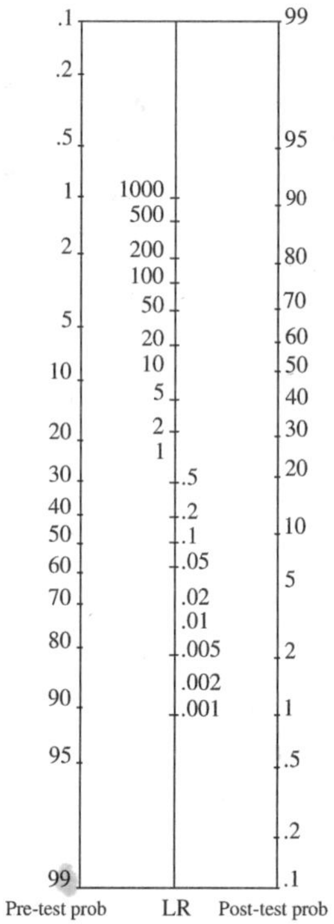

FIG. 6-1.
Likelihood ratio nomogram. (Modified from Fagan TJ. Nomogram for Bayes' theorem. *N Engl J Med* 1975; 293:257.)

Incidence

The number of patients in a given population who develop the disease over a period of time (e.g., the number of people/yr who are diagnosed with type II diabetes mellitus).

Likelihood ratio nomogram

A nomogram that allows you to calculate posttest probabilities based on pretest probability and likelihood ratio (Fig. 6-1).

Absolute risk reduction (ARR) = risk with treatment − risk without treatment

The absolute reduction in risk of having a defined adverse outcome in the treatment group compared to the control group.

Number needed to treat = 1/ARR

The number of patients who need to receive a certain treatment to achieve one additional favorable outcome.

Number needed to harm = 1/absolute risk increase (ARI)

The number of patients who, if they received a certain treatment, would lead to one additional adverse outcome compared to the patients receiving the control treatment.

7

Health Maintenance and Preventive Medicine

An apple a day keeps the doctor away . . .

INTRODUCTION

One of the major goals of outpatient medicine is to maintain the patient's health and safety and to prevent disease or detect it at a treatable stage.

RECOMMENDATIONS FOR HEALTH PROMOTION
Exercise

- All men and women should get 30–45 mins of moderate exercise at least 3–4×/wk.

Diet

- Limit fat intake to <30% total calories and saturated fat intake to <10% total calories.

- Eat 5 servings of fruits and vegetables/day.

- Include 6 servings of whole grains and fiber in the diet.

- Limit the amount of refined sugars, found in candy and soda.

- Include low-fat dairy products (2 servings/day).

Seat Belts and Helmets

- Counsel patients always to wear seat belts in the car and wear helmets if riding motorcycles or bicycles or performing such activities as inline skating.

RECOMMENDATIONS FOR DISEASE PREVENTION
Folic Acid

- For women of childbearing age who plan to become pregnant, 0.4 mg PO qd is recommended to prevent neural tube defects.

Calcium

- For men and premenopausal women, 1000 mg PO qd of elemental Ca^{2+} is recommended.

- For postmenopausal women, 1500 mg PO qd is recommended.

- Calcium carbonate (Tums, Os-Cal) contains 40% elemental Ca^{2+}/ pill and should be taken with food for increased absorption.

- Calcium citrate (21% elemental Ca^{2+}/pill) has better absorption in those with decreased stomach acidity (e.g., elderly, proton pump inhibitor therapy).

Vitamin D

- For patients >50, 200–400 IU PO qd is recommended to help prevent osteoporosis. For patients >65 or with osteoporosis, 400–800 IU PO qd is recommended. Many calcium supplements also add vitamin D.

Aspirin

- 81–325 mg PO qd is recommended for primary prevention in patients at high risk for heart disease (cardiovascular event risk >1.5%/yr) and in patients with HTN and TIAs.

- It is recommended for secondary prevention in patients with established heart disease or cerebrovascular accident.

- Enteric-coated ASA has fewer GI side effects.

Multivitamin

Consider adding a multivitamin to your patient's medications, especially if the patient has poor nutritional status.

SCREENING GUIDELINES

- Guidelines for screening differ depending on the organization recommending the guidelines. Of the major organizations setting guidelines, the *American Cancer Society* (ACS) and subspecialty societies tend to be very aggressive about screening, whereas the *American College of Physicians* (ACP) and the *U.S. Preventive Services Task Force* (USPSTF) tend to favor more conservative screening measures.

- See Table 7-1 for summarized guidelines. Note that screening needs to be **individualized** based on the patient's history and preferences.

Alcohol Abuse

- Screen periodically (see Screening for Alcoholism).

Blood Pressure

- Screen every patient q1–2yrs.

Breast Cancer

- All women should have a clinical breast exam every year.

- Screening mammograms for all women >50 q1–2yrs until age 70–75 (ACP, ACS, USPSTF).

TABLE 7-1.
SUMMARY OF HEALTH MAINTENANCE
ACTIVITIES BY AGE GROUP

Age group	Recommendations
<40 yrs	*Screening:*
	BP
	Cholesterol
	Consider DM testing for high-risk persons
	Consider HIV, STD testing
	Domestic violence screen
	For women: clinical breast exam q1–3yrs, Pap smear q1–3yrs
	Immunizations:
	Tetanus q10yrs
	Consider influenza, pneumococcal in high-risk persons
	Consider HBV in high-risk persons
	Consider varicella in high-risk persons
40–49 yrs	*Screening:*
	BP
	Cholesterol
	Diabetes testing for high-risk patients q3yrs
	Consider HIV, STD testing
	Domestic violence screen
	Colon cancer screening in high-risk patients
	For women: clinical breast exam q1–3yrs, Pap smear q1–3yrs; consider mammogram q1–2yrs
	For men: consider digital rectal exam and PSA testing q1–2yrs in high-risk patients
	Immunizations:
	Tetanus q10yrs
	Consider influenza, pneumococcal in high-risk persons
	Consider HBV in high-risk persons
	Consider varicella in high-risk persons

continued

TABLE 7-1. CONTINUED

Age group	Recommendations
50–64 yrs	*Screening:*
	BP
	Cholesterol
	Colon cancer screening
	Diabetes testing
	Consider HIV, STD testing in high-risk persons
	Consider osteoporosis screening in high-risk individuals
	Consider TSH
	Domestic violence screen
	For women: clinical breast exam q1–3yrs, mammogram q1–2yrs, Pap smear q1–3yrs
	For men: consider PSA testing q1–2yrs
	Immunizations:
	Tetanus q10yrs
	Influenza q yr
	Consider pneumococcal in high-risk persons
	Consider HBV in high-risk persons
65–75 yrs	*Screening:*
	BP
	Cholesterol
	Colon cancer screening
	Diabetes testing
	Osteoporosis screening
	Consider TSH
	Consider HIV, STD testing in high-risk individuals
	Vision, hearing, home safety screening
	Domestic violence screen
	For women: clinical breast exam q1–3yrs, mammogram q1–2yrs; consider Pap smear if not screened within past 10 yrs
	For men: consider PSA testing q1–2yrs

continued

TABLE 7-1. CONTINUED

Age group	Recommendations
	Immunizations:
	Td q10yrs
	Influenza q yr
	Pneumococcal
	Consider HBV in high-risk persons
>75 yrs	*Screening:*
	BP
	Cholesterol
	Vision, home safety, hearing screening
	Domestic violence screen
	Osteoporosis screening
	Diabetes testing
	Consider TSH
	Consider HIV, STD testing
	For women: consider clinical breast exams, mammograms, Pap smears q1–3yrs
	For men: consider PSA q1–2yrs
	Consider deferring all screening tests for cancer, particularly if patient would not want to pursue treatment.
	Immunizations:
	Td q10yrs
	Influenza q yr
	Pneumococcal
	Consider HBV in high-risk persons

- Consider screening mammograms for women age 40–49 q1–2yrs (ACS).

Cervical Cancer

- Screening Pap smears q1–3yrs for all women age 18 years, or if sexually active (ACP). High-risk groups should be screened every year; can space out to q3yrs in lower-risk populations.

- May discontinue screening >65 if prior tests have been normal (ACP, USPSTF).

Cholesterol

- Screen adults age >20 q5yrs (National Cholesterol Education Panel).

- Consider screening more frequently for those with ≥2 risk factors for coronary artery disease: family history, smoker, HTN, diabetes, high-density lipoproteins <35.

Colon Cancer

- Screen patients >50 with: (a) fecal occult blood test (FOBT) q yr or (b) flexible sigmoidoscopy q5yrs *or* (c) FOBT q yr and flexible sigmoidoscopy q5yrs *or* (d) colonoscopy q10yrs or (e) air-contrast barium enema q5yrs (ACP, ACS, USPSTF). All methods reduce mortality from colorectal cancer.

- If family history of first-degree relative with colorectal cancer or adenomatous polyps before age 60, start screening at age 40 (ACP).

Diabetes

- Not routinely indicated for healthy, asymptomatic patients (ACP).

- Consider screening with fasting blood glucose q3yrs for high-risk groups: family history, age >45, obesity, history of gestational diabetes, or of African-American, American Indian, or Hispanic descent (American Diabetes Association).

Domestic Violence

- Ask whether the patient feels as though he or she is in a dangerous situation or relationship regularly.

HIV

- Consider screening in sexually active patients with >1 partner or recent STD, homosexual or bisexual patients, IV drug users, patients who trade sex for drugs or money, and patients with history of blood transfusion from 1978–1985.

- Must do pre- and posttest counseling.

- ELISA is the screening test; Western blot is the confirmatory test.

- Do not report positive tests unless *both* the ELISA and Western blot are positive.

Osteoporosis

- Screen with DEXA scan of hip and spine all patients ≥65 and any high-risk populations: postmenopausal women not on hormone replacement therapy; women with early menopause or prolonged oligomenorrhea; and individuals with history of fragility fracture, Caucasian/Asian descent, family history of osteoporosis, and history of condition causing accelerated bone loss (corticosteroid therapy, hyperthyroidism, hyperparathyroidism) (NIH Consensus Statement, National Osteoporosis Foundation).

- Consider screening in women who are considering hormone replacement therapy, if test would facilitate decision.

- No established guidelines for screening interval.

Prostate Cancer

- Screening with prostate-screening antigen (PSA) is controversial. The recommendations range from screening all men >50 with yearly PSA and digital rectal exam (ACS) to no screening recommended (USPSTF).

- Discuss risks and benefits of screening PSA with men age >50 (ACP).

- Consider starting screening at age 40 in high-risk patients: family history of prostate cancer in first-degree relative, African-American men.

Smoking

- Screen at every visit (see Smoking Cessation).

STDs

- Screen for STDs, including chlamydia, gonorrhea, and syphilis, in patients with recent new sexual partner or multiple sexual partners, in patients with a history of STDs, in patients trading sex for money or drugs, and in all pregnant women.

- Consider routine screening in all sexually active adolescent patients and patients with a history of STDs.

- Also consider testing for HIV, hepatitis B and C in high-risk patients.

Thyroid Disease

- Screening not routinely recommended.

- Consider testing especially in patients with nonspecific symptoms (e.g., fatigue, weakness) that could be due to thyroid disease.

IMMUNIZATIONS

- See also Table 7-1.

Hepatitis A

- Two-shot series (0 and 6 mos).

- Not recommended as a routine vaccination.

- Vaccination recommended for: persons traveling to high-risk areas, food workers, hepatitis C–positive patients (to prevent decompensation of liver disease), and children.

Hepatitis B

- Three-shot series (0, 1, and 6 mos) recommended for the following: patients with >1 sexual partner or with recent STD, homosexual or bisexual patients, household contacts or sex partners of hepatitis B surface antigen–positive people, IV drug users, health care workers, hemodialysis patients, hemophiliacs, travelers to areas with high endemic rates of infection, and inmates.
- Side effects: pain at injection site, fever, Guillain-Barré syndrome (rare), anaphylaxis (rare).

Influenza

- Recommended every year for: all adults >50, all nursing home or chronic care facility patients, all adults with chronic illnesses, and all adults who may transmit influenza to high-risk populations (e.g., health care workers).
- Side effects: soreness at injection site, fever, malaise, myalgias (rare). Note that killed vaccine cannot cause influenza.

Pneumococcal Vaccine

- Recommended for: all adults >65 and adults with chronic illnesses, including diabetes, cardiovascular disease, chronic lung disease, alcoholism, liver disease, splenic dysfunction, and chronic immunosuppression (including organ transplant patients and HIV patients).
- Only one shot of the 23-valent vaccine currently available is needed if done >65; if given before then, repeat at age 65. Approximately 60% effective.
- Side effects: erythema and induration at injection site, fever and myalgias (<1%), anaphylaxis (rare).

Tetanus

- All adults should have completed a primary Td series (3 shots) and have boosters q10yrs.
- Side effects: erythema and induration at injection site, fever, Arthus reactions, anaphylaxis (rare), neurologic complications (rare).

Varicella

- Not recommended as a routine vaccination in adults due to high rate of immunity in adult population. Consider serologic testing for susceptibility if not certain of immunity status.

- Consider vaccination for patients who live or work in environments in which varicella zoster virus transmission is common: day care, schools, institutions, college dormitories, military.

- Side effects: erythema and induration at injection site, rash in <10% of patients.

What to Tell the Patient

- Screening is an important part of catching diseases at curable stages and maintaining health.

- Vaccinations can prevent morbidity and mortality from certain diseases.

- The influenza vaccine does *not* cause the flu; likewise, the pneumonia vaccine does *not* cause pneumonia.

- Discuss the expected risks and benefits of each test or immunization with the patient, as well as potential side effects, then allow the patient to make an informed decision.

Difficult Management Situations

- Some patients will decline screening tests and/or immunizations. Make sure you have discussed the risks and benefits with them, but do not force them to have a test they do not want.

- Screening is controversial in patients >75 and in patients who would not accept further workup or treatment for a positive test. Consider deferring screening tests in these patients.

OBESITY AND WEIGHT MANAGEMENT

Guidelines for Diagnosis

- The BMI measures obesity. See Table 7-2 for classification and Table 7-3 for BMI conversion table.

- BMI = weight (kg)/height (m^2).

TABLE 7-2.
WEIGHT CLASSIFICATION USING BMI

Classification	BMI	Morbidity risk
Underweight	<18.5	Low
Normal	18.5–24.9	Average
Overweight	25.0–29.9	Mild increase
Class I obesity	30.0–34.9	Moderate
Class II obesity	35.0–39.9	Severe
Class III obesity	>40.0	Very severe

TABLE 7-3.
BODY MASS INDEX (BMI) CONVERSION TABLE

BMI	19	20	21	22	23	24	25	26	27	28	29	30	35	40
Height	Weight (lbs)													
58"	91	96	100	105	110	115	119	124	129	134	138	143	167	191
59"	94	99	104	109	114	119	124	128	133	138	143	148	173	198
60"	97	102	107	112	118	123	128	133	138	143	148	153	179	204
61"	100	106	111	116	122	127	132	137	143	148	153	158	185	211
62"	104	109	115	120	126	131	136	142	147	153	158	164	191	218
63"	107	113	118	124	130	135	141	146	152	158	163	169	197	225
64"	110	116	122	128	134	140	145	151	157	163	169	174	204	232
65"	114	120	126	132	138	144	150	156	162	168	171	180	210	240
66"	118	124	130	136	142	148	155	161	167	173	179	186	215	247
67"	121	127	134	140	146	153	159	166	172	178	185	191	223	255
68"	125	131	138	144	151	158	164	171	177	184	190	197	230	262
69"	128	135	142	149	155	162	169	176	182	189	196	203	236	270
70"	132	139	146	153	160	167	174	181	188	195	202	207	243	278

continued

TABLE 7-3. CONTINUED

BMI	19	20	21	22	23	24	25	26	27	28	29	30	35	40
Height	**Weight (lbs)**													
71"	136	143	150	157	165	172	179	186	193	200	208	215	250	286
72"	140	147	154	162	169	177	184	191	199	206	213	221	258	294
73"	144	151	159	166	174	182	189	197	204	212	219	227	265	302
74"	148	155	163	171	179	186	194	202	213	218	225	233	272	311
75"	152	160	168	176	184	194	200	208	216	224	232	240	279	328

Key History

General

- Age of onset, previous weight loss experience, impact of obesity on functional status (dyspnea on exertion [DOE], resting shortness of breath [SOB], limitations on bending, lifting, moving around, energy level).

- Rule out other causes of obesity: hypothyroidism (cold intolerance, dry skin/hair, amenorrhea), Cushing's syndrome (striae, buffalo hump, symptoms of diabetes, steroid usage), polycystic ovarian syndrome (irregular menses, hirsutism).

- Ask about comorbid conditions that increase morbidity/mortality from obesity: coronary artery disease (chest pain), diabetes (polyuria, polydipsia, blurred vision), arthritis, obstructive sleep apnea (snoring, daytime somnolence).

- Ask about dietary and exercise habits: types of food, understanding of nutrition, excessive food intake, exercise program, sedentary lifestyle.

- Look for emotional stressors and history of depression and evaluate mood.

Medical History

- **Diseases** that occur at greater frequency with obesity: HTN, diabetes, coronary artery disease, osteoarthritis, gallstones, hyperlipidemia, depression/anxiety, eating disorders, cancer (colon, breast, ovary, prostate), deep venous thrombosis, gastroesophageal reflux disease, obstructive sleep apnea, cellulitis, skin abscesses, pulmonary function impairment, polycythemia

- **Medications:** Over-the-counter weight-loss medications, thyroxine, corticosteroids

- **Family history:** Obesity, coronary artery disease, diabetes, HTN

- **Social history:** Socioeconomic status, psychological stressors, tobacco abuse, alcohol abuse, social support, employment, hobbies

Focused Physical Exam

- **Vital signs:** BP, weight/height, BMI

- **HEENT:** Cataracts, deviated septum, thick neck, thyromegaly, carotid bruits, buffalo hump

- **Skin:** Striae (Cushing's syndrome), dry hair/skin (hypothyroidism), hirsutism (polycystic ovary syndrome)

- **Cardiovascular:** Displaced point of maximal impulse, left ventricular heave (long-standing HTN)

- **Pulmonary:** Decreased breath sounds

- **Abdominal:** Obesity (proportion of weight carried in the abdomen vs hips—increased abdominal obesity linked with elevated risk for comorbid conditions), masses

- **Extremities:** Range of motion of knees/hips, foot care, lower-extremity edema

- **Neurologic/psychological:** Mood

Evaluation

- **If endocrine disorders are suspected:**

  - TSH to rule out hypothyroidism

  - Dexamethasone suppression test to rule out Cushing's syndrome

- **All obese patients should be assessed for medical consequences of their obesity:**

  - Fasting blood glucose to rule out diabetes.

  - Fasting lipid panel.

  - Consider ECG/cardiac stress testing if patient complains of angina, DOE.

  - Consider sleep study if patient has symptoms of obstructive sleep apnea.

- **Before prescribing diet and exercise program or weight-loss medications:**

  - Check Chem 7, UA, and LFTs to assess renal or hepatic impairment.

Management

- **Diet, exercise, and behavior modification** are first-line therapy.

  - **Have patient keep a food diary** to record calories, fat grams, food eaten, stressors/situations in which overeating occurred.

  - **Reduce calories by 500-1000/day** to achieve weight loss of 1–2 lbs/wk. Women should choose a 1000–1200 calorie/day diet, and men should choose a 1200–1500 calorie/day diet.

  - **Nutrition education** ensures that the patient eats a balanced diet.

  - **Exercise:** Regular exercise helps weight-loss efforts, helps maintain weight significantly better than diet alone, and helps decrease risk of comorbid conditions more than diet and weight loss alone. Start with **30–45 mins of moderate exercise 3 times/wk** and build up to a daily routine.

- Keep **record of weight (inches or kg lost):**

  - Goal is to heighten awareness.

  - Proven to be one of the most helpful tools for obesity management.

- **Behavior modifications:** Eating at the table without watching television, removing all snack food from the house, laying out exercise clothes the night before as a reminder to exercise the next day.

  - **Cognitive restructuring:** Correcting negative thoughts about oneself, having realistic goals (most people only lose 5–10% of their body weight—which has an important impact on risk for comorbid conditions, but it may not be satisfactory to the patient).

  - **Stress management:** Meditation, diaphragmatic breathing, adequate social support.

- **Medications:** Should be reserved for patients with a BMI of ≥30, or a BMI of ≥27 with two comorbid conditions.

  - **Noradrenergic drugs:** Phentermine, diethylpropion, phendimetrazine. Side effects include insomnia, palpitations, tachycardia, dry mouth, dizziness, and headache.

  - **Orlistat (Xenical):** Lipase inhibitor, 120 mg PO tid with meals. Side effects include gas, diarrhea, and cramping, all of which may be severe, especially if eating a large amount of fat. **Patient may regain weight if he or she stops medication.**

  - **Sibutramine (Meridia):** Norepinephrine and serotonin reuptake inhibitor. 10 mg PO qd results in an average decrease of 5–10 lbs. Side effects include 1–3 mm Hg increase in BP, elevated heart rate, dry mouth, insomnia, constipation. **Patient may regain weight if he or she stops medication.**

  - **Gastric bypass surgery or gastroplasty** is indicated in patients with BMI ≥40 and when dietary modifications and medication therapy have failed.

When to Refer

- Patients with BMI ≥40 may be referred to weight-loss clinic for discussion about surgical options (gastroplasty and gastric bypass).

- Patients with BMI ≥27 and multiple comorbidities should be considered for enrollment in a weight-loss clinic for more intense medical management of their obesity, especially if they have failed multiple attempts at losing weight and are highly motivated.

What to Tell the Patient

- Weight management is a lifelong commitment and challenge.

- Even small amounts of weight loss can have profound impact on reduction of risk for comorbid conditions. Risk factors associated with increased morbidity and mortality in obese patients include

  - High risk of morbidity and mortality in patients with coronary artery disease, diabetes, and obstructive sleep apnea.

  - Moderate to low risk: HTN, low-density lipoprotein (LDL) >160, high-density lipoprotein (HDL) <35, age >45 (men) or >55 (women), glucose intolerance, osteoarthritis, gallstones, stress incontinence.

- Weight loss success is more likely if it is approached from all aspects: behavioral modification, diet, exercise, and medication and surgery (when appropriate).

SCREENING FOR ALCOHOLISM

Consider screening every patient as part of your social history, especially on the initial visit and periodically thereafter.

Screening Tools

- **Ask about consumption:** How many drinks do you have per day? Per week?

- Limits for **low-risk drinking:**

  - **<3 drinks/day or <7 drinks/wk for women**

  - **<4 drinks/day or <14 drinks/wk for men**

- Has alcohol ever caused a problem for you or your family?

- Do you think alcohol could be related to your current complaint?

- It may also be useful to **talk with family members** to assess the extent of the patient's alcohol use.

- **CAGE questions:**

  - Have you ever felt that you should **C**ut down on your drinking?

  - Have people **A**nnoyed you by criticizing your drinking?

  - Have you ever felt bad or **G**uilty about your drinking?

  - Have you ever had a drink first thing in the morning (an **E**ye-opener) to steady your nerves or get rid of a hangover?

Risk Assessment

- **At risk:** alcohol consumption above the recommended low-risk limits or personal or family history of alcohol-related problems.

- **Current alcohol-related problems:** CAGE score 1–2 or evidence of alcohol-related medical or behavioral problems.
- **May be alcohol dependent:** CAGE score >3 and/or 1 of the following: preoccupied with drinking, unable to stop once started drinking to avoid withdrawal symptoms, tolerance.

Interventions

Office Interventions

- **Assess the reasons** for the patient's drinking and the patient's motivation to stop drinking.
- **Advise the patient to reduce or stop drinking.** Try linking the alcohol to adverse health events, such as high BP, dyspepsia, gastritis, pancreatitis, liver disease, fetal alcohol syndrome. Alcohol-free periods of 1–2 wks may also be a good starting point.
- **Offer physician support and information about community resources,** such as Alcoholics Anonymous, National Council on Alcoholism and Drug Dependence, and psychiatric referrals if there are psychiatric issues.
- **Naltrexone (Revia),** 50 mg PO qd, or **disulfiram (Antabuse),** 500 mg PO qam, may help alcohol-dependent patients. Patients on these medications need close follow-up, however, so consider referral to a psychiatrist or an alcohol dependence program.
- **Follow up** with the patient to assess progress.

Community Resources

For the Patient

- Alcoholics Anonymous
- National Council on Alcoholism and Drug Dependence
- Outpatient day or evening treatment
- Short-term or long-term residential treatment centers

For Families

- Adult Children of Alcoholics
- Alateen—for children of alcoholics
- Al-Anon—for loved ones of alcoholics

When to Refer

Consider referral to a psychiatrist who specializes in alcohol and drug dependence for specialized treatment if the patient:

- Lacks significant social support.
- Has other drug abuse problems.
- Has symptoms of dependence.
- Has significant psychosocial issues.
- Is not safe or puts the safety of those around the patient in question.

SMOKING CESSATION

An estimated 25 million Americans smoke. Here are some tips on how to help your patient quit:

- **Ask about smoking at every visit.** Ask if your patient is interested in quitting. Educate your patient about the *risks of smoking.* Smoking has been associated with

  - **Cancer:** lung, mouth, throat, esophagus, renal cell, pancreatic, bladder
  - **Vascular diseases:** coronary artery disease, stroke, peripheral vascular disease
  - **Lung diseases:** COPD, pneumonia, asthma exacerbations in children around smokers
  - **Other diseases:** osteoporosis, macular degeneration, peptic ulcer disease, wrinkles, dental disease, low-birth-weight babies

- **Advise all smokers to quit.** Some tactics you can use:

  - **Link minor symptoms,** such as cough, sore throat, heartburn, angina, and claudication to smoking.
  - Determine the **personal benefits** your patient might gain from stopping smoking (e.g., more money in the bank, children's health) and focus on those reasons.
  - **Encourage other smokers** in the household to quit at the same time.
  - **Identify barriers to quitting** and attempt to address those problems.

- **Specific tips** to help your patient quit:

  - **Pick a quit date** together, write it in the chart, and write a prescription with the date on it to remind the patient.
  - Suggest **lifestyle changes,** such as substituting other activities when cravings occur, avoiding tempting situations and other smokers, and giving small rewards for milestones.
  - Educate the patient about **withdrawal symptoms** to expect: anxiety, difficulty concentrating, hunger, nicotine craving, depression, restlessness, insomnia.

- Offer **nicotine replacement therapy**—it doubles the quit rate.

  - **Relative contraindications:** pregnancy, nursing mother, recent MI, arrhythmias.

  - May exacerbate coronary artery disease, peptic ulcer disease, peripheral vascular disease, vasospasm, esophagitis.

  - **Nicotine gum:**

    - Dose: 1 piece q1–2h ×6 wks, then 1 piece q2–4h ×3 wks, then 1 piece q4–8h ×3 wks. Maximum, 30 pieces/day.

    - Technique: Chew gum slowly and intermittently; pause, park gum between cheek and gum to let nicotine be absorbed, and chew again until flavor released.

    - Side effects: Sore jaws, heartburn, belching, mouth irritation.

    - Cost: Around $50/box of gum.

  - **Nicotine patch:**

    - Dose: One patch (14–22 mg)/day ×6 wks, then taper.

    - Side effects: Insomnia, nightmares.

    - Cost: $20–$50/wk.

  - **Wellbutrin SR (Zyban):**

    - Dose: 150 mg PO qd ×7 days, then 150 mg PO bid ×7–12 wks—start 1 wk before quit date and take for up to 11 wks after quitting.

    - Side effects: Insomnia, dry mouth, anxiety, seizures, hypertension.

    - Cost: $100/mo.

  - **Other options** include the nicotine nasal spray and the nicotine inhaler. Both have similar effects to other nicotine products. Cost is approximately $200/mo.

- **Close follow-up** is necessary, because the majority of quitters relapse within 1 yr.

- Consider a follow-up visit and/or phone calls within the first 1–2 wks.

- Encourage relapsers to try again.

SUGGESTED READING

American Cancer Society web site. www.cancer.org/tobacco.html
American Lung Association web site. www.lungusa.org
Berke EM, Morden NE. Medical management of obesity. *Am Fam Physician* 2000;62:419–426.
U.S. Public Health Service. *Clinician's handbook of preventive services*, 2nd ed. McLean, VA: International Medical Publishing, Inc., 1997.

8 Cardiology

You've got the beat . . .

CHEST PAIN

Chest pain represents a challenge to clinicians. A systematic approach with an appreciation of the wide differential diagnosis of chest pain is the best method of beginning the evaluation (Table 8-1).

Evaluation

- **Labs:** CBC (anemia, elevated WBC with infection), electrolytes, LFTs (cholecystitis), lipid panel.

- **ECG:** A positive ECG, including ST-segment elevations, depressions, Q waves, new axis deviation, and bundle branch blocks, is concerning for ischemia/infarct and warrants urgent evaluation.

- **Chest x-ray:** Helpful in separating cardiac from pulmonic processes. Clues include cardiomegaly (cardiac disease), lung infiltrates (pneumonia), hiatal hernia (GI), widened mediastinum (aortic dissection).

- **Stress testing:** See Coronary Artery Disease.

- **2D echo:** Useful to evaluate for valvular disease and wall motion abnormalities, which indicate ischemia/infarct.

- **CT scan with contrast:** Useful for evaluation of aortic dissection.

Management

For differential diagnosis, see Table 8-1. For specific management, please see corresponding sections of this chapter.

ATRIAL FIBRILLATION

Atrial fibrillation with hemodynamic changes, ischemic changes on electrocardiography, or severe symptoms requires hospitalization!

Key History

- **General:** Fatigue or other nonspecific complaints.
- **Cardiovascular:** Palpitations, dyspnea (acute pulmonary edema).
- **Risk factors:** See Table 8-2.

Focused Physical Exam

- **Vital signs:** Increased heart rate, respiratory rate, decreased BP

TABLE 8-1.
DIFFERENTIAL DIAGNOSIS OF CHEST PAIN

Differential diagnosis	Key features
Pulmonary:	
Pneumonia	Fever, cough, pleuritic chest pain
Asthma	Dyspnea, wheezing
Pneumothorax	Dyspnea, pleuritic chest pain
Pulmonary embolism	Dyspnea, pleuritic chest pain, increased respiratory rate, increased heart rate, decreased SaO_2, clear lung exam
GI:	
GERD/hiatal hernia	Burning chest pain related to meals, sour taste in mouth
Esophogeal spasm	Severe substernal pain related to meals
Cholecystitis	Right upper quadrant abdominal/chest pain, begins after fatty meal
Dyspepsia	Nausea, vomiting, belching, bloating
Cardiovascular:	
Angina/MI	Substernal chest pressure, diaphoresis, dyspnea, nausea; related to exertion; radiation to the jaw or left arm; arrhythmia, hypotension, new murmur/congestive heart failure on exam
	Risk factors for coronary artery disease: HTN, diabetes, smoking, hyperlipidemia
Aortic dissection	Tearing sharp chest pain radiating to the back, asymmetric BP reading between arms (risk factor: HTN)
Pericarditis	Sharp substernal chest pain that increases with lying and relieved with sitting, rubbing
Musculoskeletal:	
Costochondritis	Sharp chest pain, increased with movement, reproducible
Psychiatric:	
Anxiety	Chest tightness, choking, depersonalization, feeling of impending doom

- **HEENT:** Thyromegaly
- **Pulmonary:** Rales, wheezing (pulmonary edema)
- **Cardiovascular:** Jugular venous distention/hepatojugular reflux (right heart failure). Irregularly irregular rhythm

TABLE 8-2.
RISK FACTORS FOR ATRIAL FIBRILLATION

Valvular heart disease (especially mitral stenosis)

CHF

Coronary artery disease

Hyperthyroidism

Acute pulmonary embolism

HTN

Postop (coronary artery bypass graft)

Preexcitation syndrome

COPD

Drugs: alcohol, cocaine

Medications: beta agonists, theophylline

- **Extremities:** Lower extremity edema
- **Neurologic:** Neurologic deficits (cerebral embolic event)

Evaluation

- **Labs:** Chem 7, LFTs, CBC, thyroid function tests, coagulation panel, drug screen, theophylline level (if indicated).
- **ECG:** Irregularly irregular. Absence of P waves.
- **Echocardiogram:** Valvular disease, left atrial thrombus.
- **V̇/Q̇ scan and lower extremity venous Doppler U/S or CT scan with pulmonary embolism protocol** to rule out pulmonary embolus (if clinically indicated).
- **Ischemia evaluation:** Stress echocardiography provides the benefit of the assessment of valvular function, left atrial size, and left ventricular function, as well as the assessment for ischemia. For more details on stress testing, see Coronary Artery Disease.

Management

Outpatient management is appropriate if patients are hemodynamically stable, asymptomatic, have no evidence of ischemia on ECG, and cardioversion is not planned.

Treatment strategy should center on the following:

- Ventricular rate control
- Prevention of thromboembolic events
- Restoration of normal sinus rhythm (if necessary)

Rate Control

Asymptomatic patients may be left in atrial fibrillation and started on rate-controlling medications.

- **Digoxin**

  Slow onset. Less effective than other agents. Limited in exertional rate control. Digoxin (a) does not have negative inotropic effects and (b) does have synergistic effects with other rate-controlling agents. Usual dosage: 0.125–0.5 mg PO qd. Use caution in patients with renal insufficiency.

- **Beta Blockers**

  Beta blockers are useful in patients with concomitant coronary artery disease (CAD). Bronchospasm may limit their use in patients with COPD/asthma. Cautious titration in those with congestive heart failure (CHF) due to the negative inotropic effects. The usual dosage for metoprolol (Lopressor) is 50–450 mg PO qd in divided doses and for propranolol (Inderal) is 30–640 mg PO qd in divided doses. Both are also available in extended-release formulations.

- **Calcium Channel Blockers**

  Calcium channel blockers, especially verapamil (Calan), have negative inotropic effects. Diltiazem (Cardizem) comes in a PO controlled-released formulation with a dosage of 120–360 mg PO qd. Verapamil comes in a PO slow-release formulation with a dosage of 120–480 mg PO qd.

Rhythm Control

Symptomatic patients should be chemically or electrically cardioverted. Cardioversion should be performed under the supervision of a cardiologist.

Prevention of Thromboembolic Complications

- Incidence of stroke is 5–6%; however, incidence can be up to 10–20% in elderly patients without anticoagulation. See Table 8-3 for stroke risk factors.

TABLE 8-3.
RISK FACTORS FOR STROKE IN ATRIAL FIBRILLATION

Mitral stenosis	CHF/left ventricular dysfunction
HTN	Age >65
Previous TIA or stroke	Coronary artery disease
Diabetes	

Adapted from Atrial Fibrillation Investigators. Risk factors for stroke and efficacy of antithrombotic therapy in atrial fibrillation: analysis of pooled data from five randomized controlled trials. *Arch Intern Med* 1994;154:1449–1457.

TABLE 8-4.
SUGGESTED TREATMENT STRATEGY FOR ATRIAL
FIBRILLATION PATIENTS AT RISK OF STROKE

Age	Risk factors for stroke	Therapy
<65 yrs	None	ASA or nothing (no benefit for ASA in this group)
65–75 yrs	None	ASA or warfarin (compare risk of warfarin with small risk of stroke)
Any	≥1	Warfarin (unless clear contraindication)

- **Persistent vs recurrent paroxysmal atrial fibrillation = same risk of stroke.**

- Anticoagulation should be continued *for 4 wks* after cardioversion if the patient remains in sinus rhythm. Discontinuation of anticoagulation should be determined on a case-by-case basis with the assistance of a cardiologist.

- Unless there is a direct contraindication to anticoagulation, warfarin (Coumadin) therapy should be initiated in patients with the stroke risk factors listed in Table 8-3. Table 8-4 summarizes a suggested treatment strategy.

- ASA decreases the relative risk of stroke by 25%.

- Warfarin decreases the relative risk of stroke by 60% (risk of stroke on warfarin is approximately 1%/yr).

When to Refer

Refer to a cardiologist:

- Any patient in need of chemical or electrical cardioversion

- Any patient with recurrent or sustained atrial fibrillation despite attempted chemical/electrical cardioversion and rate control that has poor tolerance of the rhythm

What to Tell the Patient

- Atrial fibrillation increases stroke risk; therefore, anticoagulation medications (ASA or warfarin) should be taken as directed.

- Monitoring of the anticoagulation level is important to prevent stroke or bleeding complications.

- Atrial fibrillation at times can be converted back to sinus rhythm; medications to convert to sinus rhythm must be taken as prescribed.

- If sinus rhythm cannot be maintained, the goal is to control heart rate and improve symptoms. Medications for rate control must be taken as prescribed. Without rate control, cardiac function can deteriorate.

- Avoid caffeine and alcohol.

CORONARY ARTERY DISEASE

- **Angina:** a syndrome resulting from myocardial ischemia.

- **Unstable angina:** (a) an accelerated pattern of angina, (b) angina at rest, (c) new-onset angina with rapidly progressive course, or (d) nocturnal angina.

- *Anyone with symptoms of unstable angina must be admitted to the hospital with telemetry monitoring.*

Classification

See Table 8-5 for Canadian Classification of Angina.

Key History

- **Cardiovascular:** Substernal tightness/heaviness, chest burning/aching, radiation to the left arm and left neck, exertional chest pain/dyspnea, palpitations

- **Pulmonary:** Shortness of breath

- **GI:** Nausea, vomiting

- **Neurologic:** Lightheadedness, diaphoresis

TABLE 8-5.
CANADIAN CLASSIFICATION OF ANGINA

Class	Definition	Example
I	No limitation with ordinary activity	Angina only with extraordinary exertion
II	Mild limitation with ordinary activity	Angina with walking >2 blocks on level surface or with climbing up >1 flight of stairs at a regular pace
III	Marked limitation with ordinary activity	Angina with walking 1–2 blocks or climbing 1 flight of stairs
IV	Unable to carry out any activity	Angina at rest or minimal exertion

From Goldman L, Hashimoto B, Cook EF, et al. Comparative reproducibility and validity of systems for assessing cardiovascular functional class: advantages of a new specific activity scale. *Circulation* 1981;64:1227–1234.

TABLE 8-6.
CORONARY ARTERY DISEASE RISK FACTORS

Male sex	Obesity
Diabetes	Smoking
Age (>45 for men, >55 for women)	Family history of premature coronary artery disease (onset <age 55)
HTN	
Hyperlipidemia (high LDL or low HDL)	

Risk Factors

See Table 8-6 for CAD risk factors.

Focused Physical Exam

- **HEENT**: Ear lobe crease, xanthelasma (hypercholesterolemia), carotid bruits
- **Pulmonary**: Rales
- **Cardiovascular**: Murmurs and gallops, especially signs of diastolic dysfunction (new-onset S_4)
- **Abdominal:** Central obesity, abdominal bruits
- **Extremities:** Diminished peripheral pulses

Evaluation

- **Lab tests:** CBC, Chem 7, LFTs, fasting lipid panel
- **ECG**
- **2D echo:** Assess for segmental/regional wall motion abnormalities, valvular disease
- **Stress testing:** A noninvasive method to assess for CAD
    - **Exercise:** Treadmill vs chemical (adenosine, dobutamine). Avoid adenosine in severe COPD or asthma.
- **Imaging:**
    - **ECG:** Positive test results include >1 mm ST depression in 2 consecutive leads, ST elevation, exercise-induced hypotension, S_3 gallop, angina. Sensitivity: 65–70%. Limitations: Specificity is poor in the presence of resting ST-T changes; difficult to interpret with left bundle branch block; ST depression does not localize the site of ischemia.
    - **Thallium or Tc Sestamibi:** Looks for areas of reversible ischemia (i.e., ischemia that reverses on rest or delayed images).

These areas are potentially viable myocardium. Ventricular size and ejection fraction can be estimated. Testing is time consuming and costly. Exercise thallium/sestamibi has a sensitivity of 80–90%, specificity of 70–90%. Adenosine thallium/sestamibi has a sensitivity of 80–90%, specificity of 70–90%.

- **Echocardiography:** Looks for improvement in segmental wall motion and thickening of the myocardial wall with low doses of dobutamine and worsening with high doses of dobutamine. These findings suggest ischemic but viable myocardium. Provides assessment of ventricular size and function and valve function. Exercise/dobutamine echo has a sensitivity of 80–90%, specificity of 80%.

Management

- **Aspirin:** ASA, 81–325 mg PO qd, reduces the rate of vascular events, including MI, in patients with stable angina.

- **Beta blockers:** Metoprolol, 25 mg PO bid; titrate to achieve goal heart rate of 60 as BP tolerates. Post MI is associated with decreased mortality. Stable angina without prior MI not associated with decreased mortality benefit; however, shown to improve symptoms.

- **Nitrates:** Sublingual nitroglycerin, 0.4 mg q5mins for chest pain. After 3 consecutive tablets, if no relief of chest pain, patient should be instructed to call 911 or go to ED. No mortality benefit in patients with CAD. Long-acting nitrates (Isordil, 10 mg PO tid, or Imdur, 30 mg PO qd) have been shown to improve symptoms and exercise tolerance.

- **ACE inhibitors:** Lisinopril (Prinivil, Zestril), 40 mg PO qd. Significant reduction in all-cause mortality, MI, stroke, and death from cardiovascular causes.

- **Lipid-lowering agents:** Simvastatin (Zocor), 20 mg PO qhs; titrate to achieve a low-density lipoprotein of <100. Lipid lowering with a statin agent reduces mortality, rate of MI, and need for coronary artery bypass graft.

When to Refer

Refer to a cardiologist for

- Patients with positive stress tests who need further evaluation with cardiac catheterization

- Patients whose symptoms are not controlled with maximal medical therapy

- Patients with arrhythmias (especially ventricular)

What to Tell the Patient

- CAD increases your risk for MI, left ventricular failure, and death.
- Controlling risk factors (HTN, diabetes, cholesterol, tobacco use) can decrease the likelihood for disease progression.
- Eating a low-calorie, low-fat/-cholesterol diet along with regular exercise also helps to decrease mortality associated with CAD.
- Take all of your medications as prescribed.
- *Chest pain that is not relieved with 3 nitroglycerin tablets must be evaluated immediately. Go to the ED or call 911.*
- Other symptoms that are cause for concern and should be evaluated promptly: new-onset chest pain at rest; chest pain increasing in severity, frequency, or intensity; worsening dyspnea; lightheadedness; syncope; dyspeptic symptoms not relieved with antacids; left arm or jaw pain.

CONGESTIVE HEART FAILURE

Etiology

See Table 8-7 for etiologies of CHF.

Key History

- **General:** See Table 8-8 for precipitants of CHF.
- **Cardiovascular:** Chest pain.
- **Pulmonary:** Shortness of breath, orthopnea, paroxysmal nocturnal dyspnea.
- **GI:** Abdominal swelling.
- **Genitourinary:** Nocturia.
- **Extremities:** Lower extremity edema.
- **Activity:** See Table 8-9 for limitations on activity.

Focused Physical Exam

- **HEENT:** Diminished carotid upstroke, bruits, presence of thyromegaly.

TABLE 8-7.
ETIOLOGIES OF CONGESTIVE HEART FAILURE

Ischemia	Cardiomyopathy
HTN	Pericardial disorders (constrictive pericarditis)
Valvular disorders	High-output failure (anemia, thyrotoxicosis)

TABLE 8-8.
PRECIPITANTS OF A CONGESTIVE HEART FAILURE EXACERBATION

Ischemia	HTN
Pulmonary embolism	Dietary noncompliance
Medication noncompliance	Myocarditis
Arrhythmia	Anemia
Infection	Pregnancy
Drugs (cocaine)	Medications (e.g., calcium channel blocker, thiazolidinediones)
Thyrotoxicosis	

- **Pulmonary:** Crackles. *The absence of crackles does not exclude elevated left-sided pressures.*
- **Cardiovascular:**
  - Right-sided failure: Jugular venous distension and hepatojugular reflux.
  - Pulmonary HTN/right ventricular strain: right ventricular heave or pulmonary artery tap.
  - Displaced point of maximal impulse, cardiomegaly, murmurs, gallops (S_3, S_4).
- **Abdominal:** Enlarged liver, venous pulsations in the liver (severe right heart failure), ascites.
- **Extremities:** Peripheral edema, tissue perfusion (peripheral pulses, skin temperature, skin color, capillary refill).

Evaluation
- **Labs:** CBC, Chem 7, LFTs, thyroid function tests, ferritin, iron panel, fasting lipid profile, troponin (if acute decompensation), urinalysis.

TABLE 8-9.
NEW YORK HEART ASSOCIATION CLASSIFICATION

Class I: No limitations with ordinary activity.
Class II: Ordinary activity results in symptoms.
Class III: Less-than-ordinary activity results in symptoms.
Class IV: Symptoms at rest.

- **ECG:** Look for strain, ischemia, low voltage.

- **2D transthoracic echocardiogram:** Assess ejection fraction, ventricular function, valve function.

- **Stress testing:** Assess for ischemic cardiomyopathy; see Coronary Artery Disease.

Management

- Attempt to identify and correct the underlying etiology of the exacerbation.

- Stress the importance of dietary and medication compliance.

- Have patients monitor their weight daily and call if weight gain exceeds 2 lbs from dry weight.

- Medication therapy:

  - **Diuretics:** The most commonly used diuretics are furosemide (Lasix), 20–320 mg PO qd in divided doses, and metolazone (Zaroxolyn), 2.5–5 mg PO qd. A synergistic effect occurs between the two if the metolazone is taken half an hour before the furosemide. Monitor potassium and magnesium levels.

  - **Digoxin:** Digoxin (Lanoxin) improves myocardial contractility. Studies have shown no improvement in mortality but a significant reduction in the number of hospitalizations for heart failure. Studies have also shown there is no benefit for doses >0.125 mg PO qd. Use with caution in patients with renal failure.

  - **ACE Inhibitors:** ACE inhibitors substantially improve morbidity and mortality among patients with heart failure. Most studies also have shown that higher doses improve mortality and reduce hospitalizations when compared to lower doses (e.g., lisinopril, 10 mg PO qd; titrate up to 40 mg PO bid as BP allows).

  - **Beta Blockers:** Should be started when patients are well compensated, not during an exacerbation. Substantially improve morbidity and mortality in patients with class II–IV heart failure (e.g., metoprolol XL [Toprol-XL], 25 mg PO qd titrated slowly up to 200 mg PO qd). Carvedilol (Coreg) and metoprolol CR/XL are currently the only beta blockers FDA-approved for the treatment of heart failure.

  - **Hydralazine/Nitrates:** The combination of hydralazine and PO nitrates has been shown to improve morbidity and mortality in patients with heart failure and can be used as an alternative regimen for patients who cannot take ACE inhibitors (e.g., hydralazine, 25 mg PO qid, titrate up to 100 mg PO qid; and isosorbide [Imdur], 30–240 mg PO qd)

- **Spironolactone:** One large study showed that there was a significant reduction in morbidity and mortality in patients with class III–IV heart failure. Dosage is 25 mg PO qd.

- **Angiotensin II Receptor Blockers (ARBs):** Losartan potassium (Cozaar), 25 mg PO qd, titrate up to 100 mg PO qd. Alternative agent for those who cannot tolerate ACE inhibitors secondary to cough. Studies comparing ARBs and ACE inhibitors have shown no significant differences between the two therapies, with the possible exception that ARBs are better tolerated.

When to Refer

Refer to a cardiologist those patients

- Who have a positive stress test and are candidates for revascularization

- Whose symptoms cannot be controlled with PO medications and are in need of IV inotropic agents or other therapies, such as left ventricular assist device or transplantation

- With arrhythmias

What to Tell the Patient

- CHF is the failure of your heart to pump blood. Blood (fluid) gets backed up and leads to edema. To reduce the risk for decompensation and admission to the hospital, you and your doctor must work together to control your disease.

- Take your medications as prescribed.

- Avoid excess sodium in your diet.

- If you are retaining fluid or gaining weight, report it to your doctor. Your doctor may ask you to take additional medicine to get rid of the extra fluid.

- A gradual exercise program is associated with improved exercise tolerance.

HYPERLIPIDEMIA

Key History

- **General:** Obesity, high-cholesterol diet, sedentary lifestyle
- **HEENT:** Hirsutism (polycystic ovarian disease)

- **Cardiovascular:** Chest pain, prior MI (CAD)

- **Medical history:** Polycystic ovarian disease, hypothyroidism, nephrotic syndrome, cholestasis or obstructive liver diseases, anorexia nervosa, diabetes, CAD, pancreatitis (from hypertriglyceridemia)

- **Social history:** Alcohol use (increased high-density lipoprotein [HDL] and triglycerides), diet, exercise

- **Family history:** History of MI, familial lipid syndromes

- **Medications:** Progestins, corticosteroids, thiazides, beta blockers

Focused Physical Exam

- **General:** Weight/BMI

- **HEENT:** Xanthelasmas, arcus corneae, thyromegaly, carotid bruits

- **GI:** Epigastric tenderness (acute pancreatitis), hepatomegaly, pulsatile mass (abdominal aortic aneurysm)

- **Extremities:** Tendon xanthomas, tuberous xanthomas, decreased peripheral pulses

Evaluation and Management

- The approach to the ambulatory patient is directed at primary and secondary prevention of hyperlipidemia.

- The National Cholesterol Education Program recommends beginning screening at age 20 (American College of Physicians recommends beginning screening in men >35 and women >45). Screening should occur yearly in those with CAD and diabetes, and q1–5yrs in all other patients.

Screening for Hyperlipidemia

- Obtain a 12-hr fasting lipid panel.

- Assess for CAD risk factors:

  - HTN

  - Diabetes

  - Family history of CAD

  - Smoking

  - HDL <40 (HDL >60 is a negative risk factor.)

  - Age (women >55, men >45)

TABLE 8-10.
TREATMENT OF HYPERLIPIDEMIA AND TARGET
LOW-DENSITY LIPOPROTEIN (LDL) LEVELS

Risk category	Start drug therapy	Lifestyle modifications	Target LDL value
0–1 risk factors	LDL >190	LDL >160	LDL <160
+2 risk factors	LDL >160	LDL >130	LDL <130
Coronary artery disease or diabetes	LDL >130	LDL >100	LDL <100

Adapted from Executive summary of the third report of the National Cholesterol Education Program (NECP) expert panel on detection, evaluation, and treatment of high blood cholesterol in adults (adult treatment panel III). *JAMA* 2001;285(19):2486–2497.

Treatment and Target LDL

See Table 8-10.

Lifestyle Modification

Lifestyle modification should always be the initial therapeutic modality, with the trial period lasting 3 mos. Patients with CAD or diabetes should begin drug therapy and lifestyle modification concurrently. Therapeutic lifestyle changes:

- Saturated fat <7% of calories, cholesterol <200 mg/day
- Soluble fiber (10–25 g/day) and plant stanols/sterols (2 g/day)
- Weight loss
- Increasing physical activity

Medications

See Table 8-11 and Fig. 8-1.

Hypertriglyceridemia

- >500 mg/dL: Reduction of triglycerides is a priority over reducing LDL. Low-fat diet (<15% of calories from fat), weight loss, and increased physical activity are important. Fibrates or niacin should be started.
- <500 mg/dL: Reduce LDL according to Table 8-11.

What to Tell the Patient

- Inform patients about specific side effects of drugs and how they can be avoided (e.g., ASA may be taken 30 mins before niacin doses to prevent flushing).

TABLE 8-11.
HYPERLIPIDEMIA MEDICATIONS

Class	LDL	HDL	TG	Adverse reactions	Contraindications
HMG-CoA reductase inhibitors	↓18–55%	↑5–15%	↓7–30%	Myopathy, increased liver enzymes	Absolute: active or chronic liver disease Relative: concomitant use of fibrate
Bile acid sequestrants	↓15–30%	↑3–5%	—	GI distress, constipation, decreased absorption of other drugs	Absolute: dysbetalipoproteinemia, TG >400 mg/dL Relative: TG >200 mg/dL
Nicotinic acid	↓5–25%	↑15–35%	↓20–50%	Flushing, hyperglycemia, hyperuricemia (or gout), upper GI distress, hepatotoxicity	Absolute: severe renal disease, severe hepatic disease
Fibric acids	↓5–20%	↑10–20%	↓20–50%	Dyspepsia, gallstones, myopathy, unexplained non-CHD deaths in WHO study	Absolute: severe renal disease, severe hepatic disease
Intestinal cholesterol absorption inhibitor	↓18%	↑1%	↓7–9%	Abdominal pain, diarrhea, fatigue, arthralgias	Absolute: severe hepatic disease. Monitor LFTs closely if used concurrently with HMG-CoA reductase inhibitor.

CHD, coronary heart disease; HDL, high-density lipoprotein; HMG-CoA, hepatic hydroxymethylglutaryl coenzyme A; LDL, low-density lipoprotein; TG, triglycerides; ↑, increased; ↓, decreased.

Adapted from Executive summary of the third report of the National Cholesterol Education Program (NECP) expert panel on detection, evaluation, and treatment of high blood cholesterol in adults (adult treatment panel III). *JAMA* 2001;285(19):2486–2497.

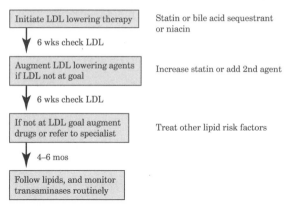

FIG. 8-1.
Hyperlipidemia treatment algorithm. [Adapted from Executive summary of the third report of the National Cholesterol Education Program (NECP) expert panel on detection, evaluation, and treatment of high blood cholesterol in adults (adult treatment panel III). *JAMA* 2001;285 (19):2486–2497.]

- Remind patients that drug therapy may be a lifelong intervention.

- Recommend exercise for patients who are physically capable. Recommendations include 45 mins of cardiovascular activity 4–6 ×/wk. Weight reduction should be reasonable (10% initially).

- Diet lists can be obtained online at the National Cholesterol Education Program web site (http://hin.nhlbi.nih.gov/ncep.htm).

HTN

Diagnosis

Category	BP
Normal	<120/80 mm Hg
Pre-HTN	120–139/80–89 mm Hg
Stage I HTN	140–159/90–99 mm Hg
Stage II HTN	160/100 mm Hg
Hypertensive urgency	Diastolic BP >120–130 mm Hg or HTN with optic disc edema or end-organ complications
Hypertensive emergency	BP >210/130 + end-organ damage (headache, blurred vision, papilledema, focal neuro deficits, chest pain, hematuria, renal failure)

Key History and Physical Exam Findings

See Table 8-12.

Evaluation

- **Labs:**

  - Chem 7 for sodium, potassium, creatinine; calcium; fasting lipid panal; hematocrit.

  - Consider TSH (for isolated systolic HTN).

  - UA to look for protein/casts, consider 24-hr urine collection for protein (if proteinuria on UA).

- **ECG:** left ventricular hypertrophy, ischemic changes

- Consider **2D echocardiogram** to assess cardiac function, particularly in patients with history of MI or congestive heart failure symptoms

TABLE 8-12.
KEY HISTORY AND PHYSICAL EXAM FINDINGS

Symptoms/signs	Suggested diagnosis
Isolated systolic HTN	Aging, thyrotoxicosis, aortic insufficiency, arteriovenous shunt, anemia
Difficult-to-control HTN	Secondary cause of HTN (see below)
Sudden increase in BP in patient with well-controlled HTN	
Sudden onset of HTN	
Age <35 at diagnosis	
Elevated serum creatinine	Renal parenchymal disease
Difficult-to-control BP, abdominal bruits	Renovascular disease, fibromuscular dysplasia (young women)
Tremor, tachycardia, heat intolerance	Thyrotoxicosis
Flushing, palpitations, labile BP	Pheochromocytoma
High BP + hypokalemia	Hyperaldosteronism
Truncal obesity, "moon facies," hyperpigmentation, hirsutism	Cushing's disease
Obesity, snoring, daytime sleepiness	Sleep apnea
Use of oral contraceptives, glucocorticoids, amphetamines, cyclosporine, NSAIDs, mineralocorticoids, decongestants, ephedra, cocaine	Drug-induced HTN

TABLE 8-13.
SECONDARY CAUSES OF HTN

Diagnosis	Diagnostic test(s)
Renovascular disease	Renal U/S with Doppler, captopril scan, MRA of renal arteries
Hyperaldosteronism	Increased serum renin/aldosterone ratio
Renal parenchymal disease	Renal U/S
Cushing's disease	Increased 24-hr urinary free cortisol
Pheochromocytoma	Increased 24-hr urinary metanephrines or plasma-free metanephrines

MRA, magnetic resonance angiography.

- Evaluation of secondary causes of HTN: see Table 8-13.

Management

- Goal BP:
  - <140/90 for patients with no comorbid conditions
  - <130/80 for patients with comorbid conditions (diabetes mellitus or CAD)
- See Table 8-14 for management protocol.
- Follow up monthly for BP checks, until BP at goal and stable, then q3-6 mos.
- Check electrolytes and renal function q6–12mos, particularly in patients on diuretics and ACE inhibitors.

TABLE 8-14.
MANAGEMENT OF HTN

Category	No cardiovascular risk factors and no end- organ disease	+ Cardiovascular risk factors but no end- organ disease	End-organ disease
Pre-HTN	Lifestyle modifications	Lifestyle modifications	Lifestyle modifications + medication
Stage I HTN	Lifestyle modifications (up to 12 mos)	Lifestyle modifications (up to 6 mos)	Lifestyle modifications + medication
Stage II or III HTN	Lifestyle modifications + medication		
HTN urgency or emergency	Consider hospital admission		

Lifestyle Modifications

- Weight loss, smoking cessation, decreased salt intake, regular exercise, decreased alcohol intake, increased K^+ and Ca^{2+} intake, stress management

Medications

See Table 8-15 for specific indications.

First Line

- Diuretics, particularly thiazides; beta blockers; ACE inhibitors

Additional Medications

- Consider adding calcium channel blockers, ARBs, clonidine.

For Refractory HTN

- Defined as failure to reach goal BP despite full doses of three drugs, including a diuretic.
- Confirm compliance with medications.
- Consider workup for secondary causes of HTN.
- Consider adding alpha blockers, minoxidil, hydralazine.

TABLE 8-15.
MEDICATION INDICATIONS/CONTRAINDICATIONS
FOR SELECTED GROUPS

Group	Medication indicated	Caution/contraindication
African-American	Thiazides, calcium channel blockers	—
Asthma/COPD	—	Beta blockers
Benign prostatic hyperplasia	Alpha blockers	—
Cerebrovascular disease	ACE inhibitors + thiazidediuretics	—
Coronary artery disease, especially post MI	Beta blockers, ACE inhibitors	—
CHF (systolic dysfunction)	ACE inhibitors ± angiotensin receptor blockers, diuretics, beta blockers, spironolactone, hydralazine/nitrates	Caution starting beta blocker during acute CHF exacerbation

continued

TABLE 8-15. CONTINUED

Group	Medication indicated	Caution/contraindication
Diabetes	ACE inhibitors, angiotensin receptor blockers	Caution with beta blockers owing to masking of hypoglycemic symptoms
Diastolic dysfunction	Calcium channel blockers	—
Gout	—	Thiazide diuretics
Hyperlipidemia	—	Thiazide diuretics
Illicit drug use, especially cocaine	—	Caution with beta blockers due to risk of unopposed alpha effects
Osteoporosis	Thiazide diuretics	—
Perioperative HTN	Beta blockers	—
Peripheral vascular disease	—	Beta blockers
Pregnancy	Methyldopa, hydralazine, labetalol	ACE inhibitors; angiotensin receptor blockers, caution with diuretics
Renal insufficiency	Loop diuretics, ACE inhibitors	—
		Caution with potassium-sparing diuretics
Renovascular disease	—	ACE inhibitors
		Angiotensin receptor blockers
Sexual dysfunction	—	Beta blockers
		Nitrates

Difficult Management Situations

- For patients with multiple comorbid conditions, see Table 8-15 for medication recommendations.

- For poorly controlled HTN, try to determine patient compliance and consider a workup for secondary HTN.

- For patients with renovascular disease:

  - Young patients with fibromuscular dysplasia benefit from renal angioplasty.

  - Elderly patients with atherosclerotic renal disease are generally treated medically first. Consider using beta blockers, ACE inhibitors,

**TABLE 8-16.
MAJOR SIDE EFFECTS OF
ANTIHYPERTENSIVE MEDICATIONS**

Class	Side effects
ACE inhibitors	Cough, angioedema, hyperkalemia
Angiotensin receptor blockers	Angioedema, allergic reaction, rash
Alpha blockers	Orthostatic hypotension, dry mouth, sedation, fatigue
Beta blockers	Bronchospasm, sexual dysfunction, masking of hypoglycemia, fatigue, depression
Calcium channel blockers	Peripheral edema, headache, dizziness
Diuretics	Thiazides: gout, pancreatitis, weakness, muscle cramps, hypokalemia, hypomagnesemia, hypercalcemia, hyperlipidemia, sexual dysfunction
	Loop: hypokalemia, hypomagnesemia, ototoxicity
	K+ sparing: hyperkalemia, gynecomastia
Vasodilators	Headache, nausea, reflex tachycardia (especially with hydralazine), orthostatic hypotension, drug-induced lupus/+ ANA (especially with hydralazine)

diuretics, and minoxidil. Surgery is indicated in patients who do not respond to medical therapy or who have worsening renal function.

When to Refer

• Patients with very difficult-to-control HTN

• Patients with secondary causes of HTN

What to Tell the Patient

• Lifestyle modifications are important. The magnitude of their effect is equivalent to one medication (up to 20 mm Hg).

• Adherence to medication regimen is very important. Most patients will require at least two medications to meet BP goals.

• End-organ damage: heart, kidneys, eyes are all affected.

• Discuss potential medication side effects (Table 8-16).

SYNCOPE

Sudden, brief loss of consciousness with loss of postural tone, followed by rapid and complete recovery, as a result of cerebral hypoperfusion.

Differential Diagnosis

Neurocardiogenic (Vasomotor Instability)

- Vasovagal (18%)
- Situational (5%): micturition, cough, deglutition, defecation
- Carotid sinus hypersensitivity (1%)
- Psychiatric disorders

Orthostatic Hypotension

- Hypovolemia (diuretics, poor intake, blood loss)
- Vasodilatation (hyperthermia, alcohol)
- Drug effects (antihypertensives, antidepressants, nitrates, opiates, sedatives)
- Autonomic insufficiency (diabetic autonomic neuropathy)

Cardiovascular

- Arrhythmias: bradyarrhythmias, tachyarrhythmias
- Anatomic/mechanical

CNS

- TIA/stroke
- Seizure (technically not syncope)
- Migraine

Key History

A thorough history is the most important means for making a reliable diagnosis. Uncovering the precipitating factor often uncovers the cause (Table 8-17).

- **Medical history:** History of syncope, cardiovascular disease, neurologic disease, HTN, diabetes, psychiatric illness
- **Social history:** Tobacco abuse, drug/alcohol abuse
- **Family history:** Hypertrophic cardiomyopathy (HCM), long QT syndrome
- **Medications:** anti-HTN, antiepileptics, antiarrhythmics, ASA

Focused Physical Exam

- **Vital signs:** Drop in systolic BP of ≥20 mm Hg 2–5 mins after standing (orthostatic hypotension), BP difference of ≥20 mm Hg between arms (subclavian steal, aortic dissection)
- **Pulmonary:** Crackles (CHF, cardiac disease)

TABLE 8-17.
SYNCOPE: PRECIPITATING FACTORS
AND SUGGESTED DIAGNOSES

Precipitating factor	Suggested diagnoses
After pain, fear, emotional distress	Vasovagal syncope
Preceded by yawning, nausea, diaphoresis	Vasovagal syncope
During coughing, micturition, defecation	Situational syncope
After standing, dehydration, antihypertensives	Orthostatic hypotension
Triggered by exertion	Aortic stenosis, hypertrophic cardiomyopathy, pulmonary HTN, pulmonary embolism, multiple sclerosis, cardiac ischemia
During shaving, head rotation, or pressure on neck	Carotid sinus hypersensitivity
Post-episode confusion, duration >5 mins	Seizure
Associated vertigo, diplopia, dysarthria	Migraine headache, TIA
Sudden loss of consciousness without warning	Arrhythmias

- **Cardiovascular:** Rate, rhythm, gallops, murmurs (cardiac disease)
- **Neurologic:** Focal neurologic deficits (TIA, migraine, structural CNS disease, seizure)

Evaluation

Initially, only history, physical exam, and ECG.

- **ECG:** Abnormal in 50% of cases, but yields diagnosis in only 5%. Perform on all patients for risk stratification. Significant findings include atrioventricular node block, bundle branch block, prolonged QT interval, left ventricular hypertrophy, and signs of prior infarction.

- Routine lab testing not recommended because it rarely yields cause—only needed to confirm or refute a diagnosis.

Key Objectives of Initial Evaluation

- Establish whether the event was actually syncope. The following are distinct clinical entities, and individuals with them should *not* be labeled as having syncope:

  - Sudden cardiac death

- Seizure: May cause loss of consciousness, but usually with prolonged recovery, postictal confusion, and/or focal neurologic symptoms. Suspect seizure if loss of consciousness >5 mins. Rhythmic jerking can occur in syncope or seizure.

- **Assign a specific cause:** Initial assessment will reveal cause without further testing in 45%.

- **Identify high-risk patients:** Even when initial assessment does not yield a diagnosis, it should identify patients with underlying heart disease, for whom more invasive and expensive diagnostic testing is indicated.

After the initial assessment, divide patients into 3 groups: diagnosis made, diagnosis suggested, or unexplained syncope.

- Diagnosis *made* on the basis of the initial assessment: treat underlying disorder without further testing.

- Diagnosis *suggested* from the initial assessment: may need specific confirmatory tests.

  - Seizure: EEG

  - Stroke or significant head trauma: neurologic imaging (head CT, MRI/magnetic resonance angiography, Doppler flow studies, and cerebral angiography)

  - Pulmonary embolism: $\dot{V}/\dot{Q}$ scan or spiral CT

  - Carotid sinus hypersensitivity: carotid sinus massage (*not recommended in patients with carotid bruits*)

  - Myocardial ischemia: exercise treadmill testing

  - Structural heart disease: echocardiography

  - Arrhythmia: ambulatory ECG (Holter) monitoring, event (loop) monitoring, implantable recorder, or electrophysiologic studies

  - Neurocardiogenic syncope: upright tilt table testing

  - Panic disorder, anxiety disorders, major depressive disorder, somatization disorder, and substance abuse/dependence: psychiatric evaluation

- *Unexplained* syncope: In the 55% of patients still undiagnosed, further testing reveals a diagnosis in approximately 50%.

Management

Vasovagal Syncope
Nonpharmacologic

- Avoid inciting factors, such as long periods of standing, dehydration, heat, fasting, and alcohol and other drugs.

- Sit or lie down immediately when symptomatic.

Pharmacologic

Usually reserved for recurrent syncope not responsive to above measures:

- Beta blockers (metoprolol, 25 mg PO bid).
- Second-line agents: fludrocortisone with increased salt intake, disopyramide, scopolamine, theophylline, ephedrine, midodrine.
- Pacemaker therapy is usually reserved for pharmacologic failure.

Cardiac Syncope

- Treat underlying anatomic disorder or arrhythmia.

Orthostatic Hypotension

- Avoid volume depletion and medications that can exacerbate orthostasis (alpha and beta blockers, vasodilators, opiates, sedatives).
- Physical interventions: Arise slowly and in stages, wear fitted stockings to reduce venous stasis, sit or lie down with any presyncopal symptoms.
- Consider pharmacologic therapy if these conservative measures fail:
  - Raise salt and fluid intake ± mineralocorticoid (e.g., fludrocortisone, 0.1–0.3 mg PO qd)
  - Other agents: alpha-1 agonists (e.g., phenylephrine, midodrine), caffeine, NSAIDs

When to Refer

- Those with unexplained syncope after history, physical exam, and ECG probably benefit from evaluation by a cardiologist.
- Those patients with cardiac syncope should be evaluated by a cardiologist.
- Hospital admission and/or telemetry monitoring criteria: known arrhythmic syncope or cardiac death, known structural heart disease, symptoms suggesting cardiac syncope, abnormal ECG, age >65.

What to Tell the Patient

- Patients with cardiac syncope have a much higher 1-yr mortality (18–36%) than do those with unexplained (6%) or noncardiac syncope (0–12%).
- There is no increase in mortality from syncope itself, but higher mortality in patients with underlying heart disease.
- Only one-third of patients with a syncopal episode will have a recurrent event in the next 3 yrs.

VALVULAR DISEASES

A murmur is a sound created by turbulent blood flow across a cardiac structure.

- **Systolic:** murmur occurring between S_1 and S_2
  - Anemia, thyrotoxicosis, sepsis, renal or hepatic failure, pregnancy, aortic/pulmonic stenosis, mitral valve prolapse, mitral/tricuspid regurgitation, HCM, atrial/ventricular septal defects
- **Diastolic:** murmur occurring between S_2 and S_1
  - Aortic/pulmonic regurgitation, mitral/tricuspid stenosis
- **Continuous**
  - Patent ductus, coarctation, arteriovenous fistula

Key History

- **HEENT:** Dental disease (risk factor for endocarditis)
- **Pulmonary:** Dyspnea, paroxysmal nocturnal dyspnea, orthopnea and edema (CHF)
- **Cardiovascular:** Chest pain, palpitations, syncope (decompensated valvular disease)
- **Medical history:** History of rheumatic fever, myocardial ischemia/infarction, congential heart diseases, murmurs
- **Social history:** IV drug use (risk factor for endocarditis)
- **Medications:** Fenfluramine (Pondimin) and dexfenfluramine (Redux) (weight-loss medications)

Focused Physical Exam

- **HEENT:** Elevated jugular venous pressure (CHF); pale conjunctiva and palmar creases (anemia)
- **Pulmonary:** Rales (CHF)
- **Cardiovascular:** Murmurs, extra sounds, heaves, thrills, displaced point of maximal impulse (Tables 8-18 and 8-19)
- **Abdominal:** Hepatojugular reflux (CHF)
- **Extremities:** Peripheral edema (CHF); cyanosis, clubbing (congenital heart disease); Roth spots, Osler's nodes, Janeway lesions (infective endocarditis)

Evaluation

- Assess the type of murmur; evaluate patient's symptoms.
- New murmurs with symptoms need prompt workup.

TABLE 8-18.
SUMMARY OF SYSTOLIC MURMURS

Systolic murmur	Type	Quality	Position	Radiation	Maneuvers	Associated findings
MR	Holosystolic	High-pitched blowing	Apex	Axilla	Squatting increases	LV heave
TR	Holosystolic	High-pitched blowing	Lower left sternum	Right sternum	Inspiration increases	Large V waves
VSD	Holosystolic	High-pitched blowing	4th–6th ICS, left sternum	—		—
AS	Ejection	Crescendo, decrescendo	2nd ICS, right sternum	Carotids	Squatting increases	Slow rise of carotid pulse
HOCM/ IHSS	Ejections	Crescendo, decrescendo	4th ICS, left sternum	—	Squatting decreases	Pulsus biferens
MVP	Midsystolic	—	Apex	—	Squatting decreases	Midsystolic click
ASD	Ejection	—	2nd ICS, left sternum	—	—	Wide fixed split S_2

AS, aortic stenosis; ASD, atrial septal defect; HOCM/IHSS, hypertrophic obstructive cardiomyopathy/idiopathic hypertrophic subaortic stenosis; ICS, intercostal space; LV, left ventricular; MR, mitral regurgitation; MVP, mitral valve prolapse; TR, tricuspid regurgitation; VSD, ventricular septal defect.

TABLE 8-19.
SUMMARY OF DIASTOLIC MURMURS

Diastolic murmur	Type	Quality	Position	Maneuvers	Associated findings
MS	Mid-diastolic	Rumble	Apex	Heard best in left lateral decubitus position	Opening snap, loud S_1, RV heave
TS	Mid-diastolic	Rumble	Xiphoid	Heard best with the bell	Opening snap
AI	Early diastolic	Decrescendo	4th ICS, left sternum	Heard best with the diaphragm	Wide pulse pressure
PI	Early diastolic	Crescendo, decrescendo	—	—	Increased with inspiration

AI, aortic insufficiency; ICS, intercostal space; MS, mitral stenosis; PI, pulmonary insufficiency; RV, right ventricular; TS, tricuspid stenosis.

- Most systolic murmurs do not represent cardiac disease and may be explained by turbulence caused by a hyperdynamic heart (e.g., anemia, renal/hepatic failure, thyrotoxicosis, pregnancy).

- Diastolic murmurs are almost always pathologic and require immediate workup.

- **Labs:** CBC, TSH, LFTs, Chem 7, and UA.

- **ECG**

- **Chest x-ray**

- **2D echocardiogram:** Easiest and most useful test to assess murmurs; should be performed in all patients with a diastolic or continuous murmur and in systolic murmurs when diagnosis cannot be made from initial evaluation or if heart failure is present.

Management and When to Refer

Aortic Stenosis

- Asymptomatic disease: evaluate yearly to assess symptoms (angina, heart failure, and syncope).

- Symptomatic aortic stenosis (patients with angina, syncope, dyspnea) should be urgently referred to a cardiologist.

- Due to the risk of hypotension, diuretics should be used cautiously and vasodilators should be avoided.

Aortic Regurgitation

- Acute aortic regurgitation caused by aortic dissection is a surgical emergency.

- Corrective surgery is indicated for symptomatic patients as opposed to long-term medical therapy.

- ACE inhibitors (lisinopril, 10–40 mg PO qd), hydralazine, and nifedipine may slow the progression of left ventricular dysfunction and delay the need for surgery.

- Stable, asymptomatic patients with chronic aortic regurgitation should follow up with a cardiologist.

Mitral Stenosis

- Echo exam is indicated to assess new symptoms and yearly to screen for increased pulmonary artery pressures.

- Negative chronotropic drugs, such as beta blockers (metoprolol, 25–100 mg PO bid) and calcium channel blockers, may be of benefit.

- Sodium restriction or diuretics (furosemide, 40 mg PO qd) for pulmonary congestion.
- Refer patients with symptomatic atrial fibrillation to a cardiologist (see Atrial Fibrillation).

Mitral Valve Prolapse

- Patients are advised to stop any stimulants, such as caffeine, alcohol, and cigarettes.
- Beta blockers (metoprolol, 25–100 mg PO bid) may reduce palpitations.

Mitral Regurgitation

- Send acute severe mitral regurgitation to ED for triage and management.
- Consider ACE inhibitors (lisinopril, 10–40 mg PO bid) for afterload reduction.
- Start diuretics (furosemide, 40 mg PO qd) for CHF.
- Refer symptomatic patients to cardiology.

Tricuspid Valve Regurgitation

- Echocardiography can be used to characterize the etiology, as tricuspid valve regurgitation may accompany severe mitral stenosis and pulmonary HTN.

Hypertrophic Cardiomyopathy

- A genetic disease characterized by hypertrophy of the left ventricle—typically autosomal-dominant pattern of inheritance.
- Complications include sudden death, CHF, arrhythmias, and infective endocarditis.
- Medical therapy includes beta blockade (metoprolol, 25–100 mg PO bid). Use calcium channel blockers with caution.
- Avoid digitalis, diuretics, nitrates, and beta-agonists.
- Refer to cardiology for additional evaluation and surveillance.

Antibiotic Prophylaxis

- Endocarditis prophylaxis for dental or oral procedures is indicated for moderate and high-risk valvular diseases (Table 8-20).
- Initiate antibiotics shortly before a procedure and no more than 6–8 hrs after a procedure.
  - Amoxicillin, 2 g PO ×1, 1 hr before procedure.

TABLE 8-20.
AMERICAN HEART ASSOCIATION RECOMMENDATIONS
FOR PREVENTION OF BACTERIAL ENDOCARDITIS

High risk	Moderate risk	Low risk
Prosthetic valves	PDA	Innocent heart murmurs
History of IE	VSD/ASD	MVP with normal echo
Cyanotic congenital heart disease	Coarctation	and no regurgitation
	Bicuspid AV	
Surgically constructed conduits	RHD/CVD	
	HOCM	
MVP with regurgitation	MVP with thickened leaflets	

AV, aortic valve; HOCM, hypertrophic obstructive cardiomyopathy; IE, infectious endocarditis; MVP, mitral valve prolapse; PDA, patent ductus arteriosis; RHD/CVD, rheumatic heart disease/cerebrovascular disease; VSD/ASD, ventricular septal defect/atrial septal defect.
Adapted from Dajani AS, Taubert KA, et al. Prevention of bacterial endocarditis. Recommendations by the American Heart Association. *JAMA* 1997;277:1794–1801.

- Penicillin allergy: clindamycin, 600 PO mg; cephalexin or cefadroxil, 2 g; or azithromycin, 500 mg PO ×1, 1 hr before procedure.
- If the patient cannot tolerate PO: ampicillin 2 g IV, 30 mins before procedure, or clindamycin, 600 mg IV, or cefazolin, 1 g IV, 30 mins before procedure.

Rheumatic Heart Disease
- Primary prevention involves identifying and treating upper respiratory infections caused by group A *Streptococcus*.
- Secondary prevention involves treating patients with rheumatic fever history. Treatment involves penicillin V, 250 mg PO bid, or erythromycin, 250 mg PO bid.

Anticoagulation
See Table 8-21.

What to Tell the Patient
- Statistically speaking, most murmurs are benign and stable.
- Reassure patients and instruct them to return to the office if symptoms develop.

TABLE 8-21.
ANTICOAGULATION FOR VALVULAR
DISEASES/VALVE REPLACEMENT

Valve	Anticoagulation
Tissue valve	Coumadin target INR of 2–3 for 3 mos, then ASA 325 mg PO qd lifelong
Mechanical valve	Coumadin target INR of 2.5–3.5 lifelong
St. Jude's valve in the aortic position	Coumadin target INR of 2–3 lifelong
MVP with focal neurologic events	ASA 81–325 mg PO qd
MVP in association with previous CVA, recurrent TIA, AF, and age >65, MR, HTN, or heart failure history	Coumadin target INR of 2–3

AF, atrial fibrillation; CVA, cerebrovascular accident; MR, mitral regurgitation; MVP, mitral valve prolapse.
Adapted from Bonow RO, Carabello B, et al. Guidelines for the management of patients with valvular heart disease. *Circulation* 1998;98:1949–1984.

- Depending on the type of valvular disease, some patients may need antibiotic prophylaxis before procedures.

SUGGESTED READING

Bonow RO, Carabello B, et al. Guidelines for the management of patients with valvular heart disease. *Circulation* 1998;98:1949–1984.

Chobanian AV, Bakris GL, Black HR, et al. The seventh report of the Joint National Committee on Prevention, Evaluation, and Treatment of High Blood Pressure: the JNC-7 Report. *JAMA* 2003;289(19):2560–2572.

Dajani AS, Taubert KA, et al. Prevention of bacterial endocarditis. Recommendations by the American Heart Association. *JAMA* 1997; 277:1794.

Epstein AE, Vidaillet H, et al. Frequency of symptomatic atrial fibrillation in patients enrolled in the Atrial Fibrillation Follow-Up Investigation of Rhythm Management (AFFIRM) study. *Cardiovasc Electrophysiol J* 2002;13(7):667–671.

Executive summary of the third report of the National Cholesterol Education Program (NECP) expert panel on detection, evaluation, and treatment of high blood cholesterol in adults (adult treatment panel III). *JAMA* 2001;285(19):2486–2497.

Falk RH. Medical progress: atrial fibrillation. *N Engl J Med* 2001;344: 1067–1078.

Heaven DJ, Sutton R. Syncope. *Crit Care Med* 2000;28:N116–N120.

Kapoor WN. Syncope. *N Engl J Med* 2000;343:1856–1862.

Linzer M, Yang EH, et al. Diagnosing syncope. Part 1: Value of history, physical examination, and electrocardiography. Clinical Efficacy Assessment Project of the American College of Physicians. *Ann Intern Med* 1997;126:989–996.

Linzer M, Yang EH, et al. Diagnosing syncope. Part 2: Unexplained syncope. Clinical Efficacy Assessment Project of the American College of Physicians. *Ann Intern Med* 1997;127:76–86.

Dermatology

And by the way, I've got this rash . . .

APPROACH TO SKIN DISEASES
Key History
Skin:

- Characteristics of initial lesion
- Duration of lesion
- Evolution of lesion
- Symptoms, including pruritus, erythema, drainage
- Recent contacts (hobbies, outdoor activities)
- Recent changes in diet, detergents, cosmetics
- Exacerbating and relieving factors

Medical history:

- Asthma (atopy)
- Systemic diseases (SLE, vasculitis, thyroid disease, malignancy, inflammatory bowel diseases, sarcoidosis, syphilis, infections)
- Pregnancy
- CNS disease
- HIV

Family history: Atopy, psoriasis

Social history:

- Relationship of lesion to travel history, drug ingestion, recent contacts, occupation, hobbies, heat/cold, treatments, changes in diet/detergents/cosmetics

Focused Physical Exam

Examine entire skin surface, including scalp, mucous membranes, and nails. Ensure adequate illumination; side lighting helps to identify subtle elevated lesions. Important characteristics to identify:

- **Location(s)** of lesion
- **Morphology** of lesion:
  - *Macule*: Flat lesion <1 cm

- Patch: Flat lesion >1 cm (slight scale or fine wrinkling)
- Papule: Elevated skin lesion <5 mm diameter
- Plaque: Elevated flat lesion >5 mm diameter
- Nodule: Elevated skin lesion >5 mm diameter
- Cyst: Nodule filled with liquid or semisolid material
- Vesicle: Blister filled with clear fluid, <5 mm diameter
- Bulla: Blister filled with clear fluid, >5 mm diameter
- Pustule: Vesicle filled with purulent fluid
- **Color of lesion:** Erythematous, hypopigmented, hyperpigmented
- **Other descriptors:** Crust, scale, lichenification, induration, fissure, erosion, ulcer, atrophy, wheal, telangiectasia
- **Configuration of lesions:** Individual, grouped, linear, follicle centered
- **Palpation:** Consistency, mobility, tenderness, depth
- **Margination:** Well or ill defined, flat or raised
- **Epidermal and/or dermal** involvement

Evaluation

- **Microscopic exam:**
  - Scale: potassium hydroxide (KOH) preparation (fungus)
  - Pustule: Gram stain, culture
  - Vesicle: Tzanck preparation (herpes simplex virus)
  - Burrows: exam for scabies mite
- **Wood's lamp exam** (fungal infections)
- **Biopsy** (shave or punch) for unknown lesion or if suspicious of skin malignancy. Do not do a shave or punch biopsy if malignant melanoma is suspected; an excisional biopsy is required.
- **Patch tests**
- **Labs** with suspicion of systemic disease (i.e., CBC, ANA, VDRL, ESR, rheumatoid factor)
- **X-rays** with suspicion of systemic disease (e.g., sarcoidosis)

Management

Depends on underlying condition (see specific diagnoses for treatment options).

ACNE VULGARIS

Inflammation of the pilosebaceous units of the skin. There are three types of acne: comedonal, papulopustular, and nodulocystic.

Key History

- **Skin:** Pustular, comedonal, or nodular lesions on the face and trunk with a duration of weeks to months. Symptoms may be worse in fall and winter.

- **Medical history:** Polycystic ovarian syndrome (PCOS)

- **Medications:** Androgenic steroids (particularly in athletes), lithium, corticosteroids

Focused Physical Exam

- **Comedones:** Open, dilated pores filled with black keratinous material (blackheads) or closed, skin-colored papules (whiteheads).

- **Papules and pustules:** With or without inflammation (erythema) and crusting.

- **Nodules:** 1–4 cm diameter, erythematous. Subsequent scars may be depressed or hypertrophic.

- Lesions may be isolated or scattered on the face, neck, upper arms, trunk, and buttocks.

Evaluation

Generally, history and physical exam are sufficient to make the diagnosis.

- **Labs:** In women in whom you suspect PCOS, draw a free testosterone level (>200 mg/dL suggestive of PCOS), follicle-stimulating hormone and luteinizing hormone (luteinizing hormone:follicle-stimulating hormone ratio of > 3:1 is suggestive of PCOS), and DHEA-S (increased in PCOS).

- In most women with acne, the hormone levels will be normal.

Management

Mild Acne (Comedonal or Papulopustular)
Topical Antibiotics

- Clindamycin, 1% (Cleocin T) bid, or erythromycin, 2% bid, or benzoyl peroxide, 2, 5, or 10% qd–bid

- Side effects: Burning, itching, dry skin, peeling

Topical Retinoids

- Particularly effective for comedonal acne. Patients should apply at night and wait 20 mins after washing face to apply medication (owing to drying effects).

- Tretinoin (Retin-A): Start with 0.025% cream or 0.01% gel; can titrate to 0.05% cream or 0.025% gel. If still no response, try 0.1% cream or 0.05% liquid. Apply to face qhs.

- Adapalene (Differin), 0.1% qhs.

- Side effects: Peeling, erythema, blistering.

Moderate Acne (Papulopustular)

- Add PO antibiotics (tetracycline, 500 mg PO bid; erythromycin, 500 mg PO bid; doxycycline, 100 mg PO bid; or minocycline, 100 mg PO bid) to the topical regimen.

- Oral estrogens combined with progesterone (i.e., oral contraceptives) may be useful in females.

Severe Acne

- Isotretinoin (Accutane), 1 mg/kg/day PO divided bid × 15–20 wks. May be repeated if necessary.

- Side effects: dry mouth, lips, eyes; night blindness; contact lens irritation; eczema-like rashes; elevated triglycerides; decreased high-density lipoprotein; elevated cholesterol; hepatotoxicity; depression (some case reports of suicide as well).

- Monitor LFTs q4–6wks and pregnancy tests q4wks.

- **Highly teratogenic**—women must have a negative pregnancy test before beginning therapy and must be on a **reliable birth control method** while being treated!

When to Refer

Refer to dermatology for severe or refractory cases.

What to Tell the Patient

- Emotional stress may exacerbate acne.

- Occlusion and pressure on skin by resting the face on hands or a telephone can exacerbate acne.

- Acne is *not* caused by chocolate or fatty foods, or any other type of food.

- Topical preparations may irritate the skin, so the acne may first appear to worsen with treatment due in part to skin irritation.

- Topical preparations should be applied to the entire area, not just individual lesions.

- Picking or "popping" acne may cause skin damage and subsequent scarring.

ACNE ROSACEA

Inflammation of the skin characterized by papules, pustules, and telangiectasias. Occurs most often in adults, with onset usually between 30 and 50 yrs, with a female predominance.

Key History

- **Skin:** Facial flushing and warmth exacerbated by hot drinks, alcohol, and sun exposure
- **HEENT:** Red eyes, eyelid inflammation, and swelling (blepharitis)
- **Medications:** ACE inhibitors, vasodilators, simvastatin (Zocor)

Focused Physical Exam

- **Skin:** Facial erythema, papules, pustules, telangiectasias, skin thickening (cheeks, chin, nose)
- **HEENT:** Conjunctival injection, eyelid swelling, chalazia

Evaluation

Generally a clinical diagnosis made by history and physical exam.

Management

Lifestyle Modifications

- Avoid triggers (alcohol, hot drinks, excessive sun exposure).
- Avoid harsh, drying soaps; mild, nondrying soaps are recommended.

Topical Therapy

- Metronidazole gel, 0.75% bid to affected areas for mild cases.

Systemic Antibiotics

- Tetracycline, 250 mg PO qid, until symptoms controlled.
- For severe or resistant cases, minocycline, 50–100 mg PO qd, or isotretinoin, 0.5–1 mg/kg/day for 15–20 wks are options.

When to Refer

- Refer to dermatology for severe or refractory cases.

What to Tell the Patient

- Rosacea is a chronic skin condition that is recurrent; the cause is unknown, and it is not related to poor skin hygiene.
- Lifestyle changes are important in avoiding episodes of rosacea.

CONTACT DERMATITIS

- Inflammatory response of skin to an external chemical. Can be caused by an irritant or allergic reaction.

Key History

Risk Factors for Contact Dermatitis

- Outdoor activities with potential contact with poison ivy, poison sumac, poison oak
- Recent changes in soaps, detergents, fabrics, cosmetics
- Skin exposure to nickel (in watches, jewelry)
- Exposure to latex rubber
- Exposure to topical medications (e.g., neomycin, topical "triple antibiotic" cream)
- History of allergies, atopy

Focused Physical Exam

- Erythematous rash.
- Vesicles may or may not be present (acute).
- Lichenification (chronic).
- Lesion configuration and location (may provide additional clues to the underlying irritant).

Evaluation

- History and physical exam are usually enough to identify a causative agent and establish the diagnosis.
- Consider patch testing to help identify potential causative agents in allergic contact dermatitis.

Management

Identifying the irritant is crucial so that future contact can be avoided or minimized with protective clothing.

Topical Steroids

- Triamcinolone, 0.025% bid, or hydrocortisone, 1% or 2.5% bid–qid.
- Avoid high-potency steroids on face, ears, and penis; can cause skin atrophy and telangiectasias.

Systemic Antihistamines

Helpful for pruritus:

- Diphenhydramine (Benadryl), 25 mg PO q6h

- Fexofenadine (Allegra), 180 mg PO qd

- Loratadine (Claritin), 10 mg PO qd

- Cetirizine (Zyrtec), 5–10 mg PO qd

Severe dermatitis may require a short course of **systemic steroids** (prednisone, 40–60 mg PO qd × 5 days, then taper, or triamcinolone [Kenalog-40] IM). Aveeno (1 packet/bath qd) may improve weeping and itching.

When to Refer

- Refer to a dermatologist for biopsy in cases in which the diagnosis is not clear or for very severe cases refractory to treatment.

- Refer to an allergist for skin patch testing if needed to identify the irritant.

What to Tell the Patient

- It is important to identify and avoid the offending agent when possible.

- Avoid scratching, which may leave scars.

ATOPIC DERMATITIS

Chronic, pruritic eczematous dermatitis associated with a personal or family history of atopy (allergic rhinitis, asthma, or atopic dermatitis). Often exacerbated by foods, changes in climate, emotions, etc.

Key History

- **General:** Pruritus

- **Skin:** Rash (face, neck, upper chest, antecubital/popliteal fossa), often recurrent and worse with hot weather

- **Medical history:** Allergic rhinitis, asthma, Churg-Strauss syndrome

- **Family history:** Allergic rhinitis, asthma, atopic dermatitis

Focused Physical Exam

- Erythematous patches with papules, vesicles, and crusting

- Lichenification and scaling (chronic)

- Dry skin

- Facial erythema

- Increased linear markings on palms

Evaluation

- Diagnosis is made clinically.

- Skin testing may be useful to identify sources of irritation.

Management

- **Nonpharmacologic treatment:** Cold compresses, moisturizers, and Aveeno (1 packet/bath) can help with pruritus.

- **Topical steroids** are the mainstay of treatment.

  - Start with a medium-potency steroid (e.g., triamcinolone, 0.5% bid).

  - Can increase steroid potency if necessary. Use caution with sensitive areas, especially on face (can cause skin atrophy); intermittent use only.

- **Tacrolimus:**

  - Apply 0.1% ointment bid for moderate to severe dermatitis unresponsive to topical steroids.

  - Side effects: Skin burning/tingling, pruritus, skin infections (herpes simplex virus, folliculitis).

- **Systemic antihistamines** are useful particularly for pruritus (e.g., fexofenadine [Allegra], 180 mg PO qd, or cetirizine [Zyrtec], 5–10 mg PO qd).

- **Antibiotics** are indicated for skin infections; cover for *Staphylococcus* and *Streptococcus* species with cephalexin, 500 mg PO q6h, or dicloxacillin, 500 mg PO q6h.

- **Systemic steroids** may be used to bring severe disease under control (e.g., prednisone, 10–60 mg PO qd, taper as quickly as possible to minimize side effects).

When to Refer

Refer to dermatology for severe or difficult-to-manage atopic dermatitis. Additional therapies (ultraviolet B, PUVA, immunomodulants, tacrolimus) may be used.

What to Tell the Patient

- Atopic dermatitis is a chronic disease with acute flares and long recoveries.

- It is important to reduce exposure to known irritants and avoid scratching.

SEBORRHEIC DERMATITIS

Chronic, superficial, inflammatory disease affecting the scalp, eyebrows, and face.

Key History

- **Skin:**

  - Dry, flaky, greasy patches of skin

- Pruritus

- Seasonal variation: often improves in summer owing to increase in ultraviolet light exposure, flares in the fall/winter (decreased sunlight)

- **Medical history:** HIV (seborrheic dermatitis is common in patients with HIV), CNS disease

Focused Physical Exam

Skin:

- Erythematous, symmetric patches and plaques with yellowish, greasy scale in areas with numerous sebaceous glands (i.e., hairy areas).

- Common areas include scalp, eyebrows, eyelids, ears, nasolabial folds, chest, intertriginous areas, axilla, groin, buttocks, and inframammary folds.

Evaluation

Diagnosis is usually made from history and physical exam.

Management

- Initiate treatment with shampoos (zinc pyrithione [DHS Zinc, Head and Shoulders] 1%, selenium sulfide [Exsel, Head and Shoulders Intensive Treatment Dandruff Shampoo, Selsun, Selsun Blue] 1% or 2.5%, or ketoconazole [Nizoral] 1% or 2%) 2–3 times/wk. Rub shampoo onto wet scalp, rinse, and reapply. After 3–5 mins, perform final rinse.

- Use a topical steroid lotion or gel in nonhairy areas. Hydrocortisone cream (1% or 2.5%) or ketoconazole cream, 2% bid, may be used as needed.

What to Tell the Patient

- Seborrheic dermatitis is a chronic disease that can be well controlled with regular use of the shampoos listed above.

- It is a common problem affecting 3–5% of the population.

STASIS DERMATITIS

- Occurs on the lower legs of patients with peripheral vascular disease.

- Pathophysiology: venous incompetence causes increased hydrostatic pressure leading to capillary damage and extravasation of blood and resulting in inflammation.

Key History

Skin: Edema and swelling of the lower legs with development of a chronic, pruritic eruption.

Focused Physical Exam
Skin:

- Hyperpigmented or erythematous thickened skin with scale and weeping.
- Varicose veins may be prominent.
- The most common site of involvement is above the medial malleolus.

Evaluation

The diagnosis is made clinically.

Management

- The prevention of venous stasis and lower extremity edema is imperative for effective management of stasis dermatitis.
- Support stockings (e.g., TED hose), weight reduction, and leg elevation at rest may be effective.
- Lesions are treated with topical steroids (e.g., triamcinolone, 0.1% bid–tid) and wet compresses (for weeping areas).

What to Tell the Patient

- It is important to prevent stasis and edema.
- To help prevent stasis dermatitis, consistent leg elevation and use of support stockings are important.

TINEA

Fungal infection of the epidermis.

Key History
Skin:

- Scaling rash, pruritus, hair loss.
- Can occur in several places through the body (see below).

Focused Physical Exam
Skin:

- **Scalp** (tinea capitis): Erythematous patches and plaques with scale; patchy alopecia and broken hair shafts; indurated, boggy plaques; crusting; pustules; and scarring.
- **Face** (tinea faciale): Erythematous patches and plaques with minimal scale.
- **Body** (tinea corporis): Annular, erythematous patches and plaques with scale; may have central clearing.

- **Hand** (tinea manuum): Diffuse, dry scaling. Usually only on one palm.

- **Groin** (tinea cruris): Erythematous patches or plaques with elevated, scaling, well-marginated, and serpiginous borders. Weeping, maceration, and pustules may be present.

- **Feet** (tinea pedis): Diffuse scaling on soles and sides of feet ("moccasin distribution"), interdigital maceration (most commonly between fourth and fifth toes), or vesicles and pustules on instep.

- **Trunk** (tinea versicolor): White, pink, or tan (usually hypopigmented) patches with fine scale.

- **Nails** (onychomycosis): Yellow, flaking, split nails.

Evaluation

- **Potassium hydroxide (KOH) preparation** (see Chap. 25, Procedures): presence of hyphae on KOH preparation is diagnostic of a dermatophytic or candidal infection.

- **Fungal culture:** Can be done for patients with a high clinical suspicion of dermatophyte infection but a negative KOH preparation.

Management

Topical antifungals are the treatment of choice for most dermatophyte infections. The exceptions are tinea capitis (treatment described below) and onychomycosis.

- Initial topical therapy includes imidazole creams (clotrimazole, 1%; miconazole, 2%) bid.

- Other options include naftifine, 1%; terbinafine, 1% qd; or ciclopirox, 1% bid.

- Chronic tinea pedis infection may require suppressive therapy with miconazole powder qd.

- Patients with widespread disease or disease refractory to topical therapy may require systemic therapy.

For **tinea capitis,** topical agents are ineffective.

- Griseofulvin, 500 mg PO qd (microsized type), or 375 mg PO qd (ultramicrosized type) × 4–6 wks and selenium sulfide shampoo 2×/wk.

- If oral griseofulvin fails, terbinafine (250 mg PO qd × 4–6 wks), ketoconazole (200 mg PO qd × 4–6 wks), or itraconazole (Sporanox) (200 mg PO qd × 4–6 wks) is recommended.

- Oral prednisone (1 mg/kg/day) may be given with systemic antifungals to help reduce the incidence of scarring in markedly inflammatory tinea capitis.

For **onychomycosis,** PO antifungals are necessary for effective treatment. As these treatments are expensive and have potentially dangerous side effects, diagnosis should be confirmed before starting treatment.

- Itraconazole (Sporanox) "pulse dosing": 200 mg PO bid for first week of month × 2 mos (fingernails) or 3–4 mos (toenails). Monitor LFTs while on medication.

- Terbinafine (Lamisil), 250 mg PO qd × 6 wks or 500 mg PO qd for first week of month × 2 mos (fingernails) or 4 mos (toenails). Monitor LFTs while on medication.

When to Refer

Refer to dermatology for severe infections or infections with poor response to topical antifungals.

What to Tell the Patient

- The incidence of dermatophytic infections is higher in warmer, humid climates.

- Treatment with topical antifungals is usually sufficient.

- Chronic or recurrent infections may require changes in personal hygiene.

WARTS

The common wart is caused by papillomavirus infection (commonly, HPV types 2, 4, 27, and 29) of epidermal cells.

Key History

- **Skin:** Warts usually begin unnoticed and gradually grow.

- **Medical history:** Immunosuppression.

Focused Physical Exam

Skin: Skin-colored, firm papules or nodules with hyperkeratotic surfaces that interrupt the normal skin lines and may be studded with black puncta, usually on hands, fingers, and sole of foot.

Evaluation

Usually a clinical diagnosis.

Management

Warts commonly remit within 2 yrs, especially in children, so no treatment may be necessary. Treatment options include

- Topical salicylic acid preparations can be found over the counter and can be effective in treating warts.

- Liquid nitrogen (cryosurgery) is commonly used. Apply liquid nitrogen with cotton-tipped applicator or spray to wart plus 2 mm of surrounding tissue for 30 secs. May need to be repeated q2wks until wart is gone.
- For refractory warts, refer to a dermatologist for electrodessiccation and curettage, surgical excision, or laser therapy.

When to Refer
Referral to a dermatologist may be useful for treatment of multiple lesions or lesions refractory to standard therapy, or further workup of suspected carcinoma.

What to Tell the Patient
- Common warts are common.
- To cure a wart, *all* infected cells must be destroyed. Therefore, shaving or "picking" off a wart does not eradicate the infection.
- Multiple treatments may be required.

URTICARIA

Key History
- **Skin:**
  - Eruptions of hives lasting a few hours, then disappearing.
  - May be pressure, sun, cold, stress, or exercise induced.
  - Exposure to new lotions, soaps, cosmetics, laundry detergents, perfumes.
- **Medical history:** Atopy (allergies, asthma), food allergies, SLE, thyroid disease, polycythemia vera, angioedema
- **Medications:** All medications, particularly new medications (penicillin, sulfa, ACE inhibitors, ASA)
- **Social history:** Diet (shellfish, eggs, strawberries, nuts, tomatoes, etc.) eaten in last 24 hrs

Focused Physical Exam
Skin: Erythematous, annular plaques with central pallor and changes in size and shape over time

Evaluation
- Try to identify the offending agent.
- For acute urticaria with likely etiology identified, no further workup is necessary.

- Labs: CBC with eosinophil count.

- Consider ANA, TSH, ESR, LFTs if indicated by history or physical exam.

- Consider skin testing or RAST (radioallergosorbent test, which measures allergen-specific IgE) testing for offending agents. Skin testing is more sensitive and specific, but RAST testing is indicated in patients with dermatographism or in whom skin testing may be dangerous (e.g., history of anaphylactic reaction).

- Consider referral for skin biopsy if diagnosis is unclear.

Management

- **Avoidance of triggers.** If a food allergy is suspected, have the patient restrict diet (e.g., eliminate common sources of allergy, including nuts, eggs, shellfish, tomatoes, yeast) and keep a food and symptom diary. Stop or substitute any suspected medications.

- **PO antihistamines** are first-line therapy: loratadine, 10 mg PO qd; fexofenadine, 180 mg PO qd; or cetirizine, 10 mg PO qd.

- **Systemic corticosteroids** (prednisone, 40–60 mg PO qd) may be necessary for severe eruptions.

When to Refer

- Refer to dermatology for biopsy if the diagnosis is unclear.

- Refer to allergist for skin and/or RAST testing.

What to Tell the Patient

- Urticaria is common and can usually be controlled by eliminating the offending agent.

- Avoidance of triggers is important in controlling eruptions.

SUGGESTED READING

Fitzpatrick TB, Eisen AE, et al., eds. *Dermatology in general medicine.* New York: McGraw-Hill, 1993:489–514.

Fitzpatrick TB, Johnson RA, et al. *Color atlas and synopsis of clinical dermatology*, 3rd ed. New York: McGraw-Hill, 1997:2–7, 48–63, 72–74, 76–91, 688–717, 766–771.

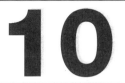# Endocrinology

Hormones running wild . . .

DIABETES MELLITUS

The following section focuses on the outpatient management of type II diabetes.

Classification

- Type I: Autoimmune disorder resulting in destruction of the beta cells of the pancreas. Patients usually present in childhood, are insulin dependent, and are at risk for diabetic ketoacidosis (DKA). 10% of all diabetics.

- Type II: Insulin resistance accompanied by impaired insulin secretion. Commonly presents in obese adults. May or may not be insulin dependent. 90% of all diabetics.

Complications

Acute

- Hyperglycemia
- Hypoglycemia
- DKA (seen in type I)
- Hyperosmolar coma syndrome (seen in type II)

Chronic

- Microvascular: neuropathy, nephropathy, retinopathy
- Macrovascular: HTN, CAD, cerebrovascular disease, peripheral vascular disease (PVD)

Key History

- **General:** Fatigue, weakness or classical complaints of polyuria, polyphagia, polydipsia, and blurred vision (hyperglycemia); diaphoresis (hypoglycemia)
- **HEENT:** Vision change or loss (retinopathy)
- **Cardiovascular:** Angina (CAD), palpitations (hypoglycemia)
- **GI:** Diarrhea, nausea/vomiting, early satiety (autonomic neuropathy)
- **Genitourinary:** Vaginal discharge (candidiasis)
- **Extremities:** Claudication (PVD), foot ulcers, toe amputations

- **Neurologic:** Weakness/numbness/burning in the extremities (peripheral neuropathy), tremor (hypoglycemia)
- **Medical history:** Obesity, polycystic ovary syndrome, gestational diabetes, hypertriglyceridemia
- **Family history:** Family history
- **Medications:** Steroid use, current diabetes treatment (diet, oral agents, insulin)

Focused Physical Exam

- **Vital signs:** BP, weight
- **HEENT:** Proliferative retinopathy and macular edema (diabetic retinopathy)
- **Extremities:** Diminished distal pulses (PVD), peripheral/periorbital edema (nephrotic syndrome), foot ulcers/calluses
- **Neurologic:** Diminished light touch and vibratory sensation in feet (peripheral neuropathy), weakness, absent reflexes (mononeuropathy)
- **Skin:** Hyperpigmented lesion in the axilla or on the nape of the neck (acanthosis nigricans), shiny atrophic lesion on the legs (necrobiosis lipoidica diabeticorum)

Evaluation

- **Diagnosis of diabetes:**
  - (a) Classic symptoms of diabetes *and* random blood sugar >200 mg/dL or
  - (b) Fasting blood sugar of >126 mg/dL
- **Blood sugar monitoring:** Equip patients with a home glucometer and instruct them in its usage. Patients should monitor blood glucose 2–3×/day and should record results to bring with them to each clinic visit. Check HgbA1c q3–6mos.
- **Renal monitoring:** Patients should have annual urine dipstick monitoring to evaluate for the development of proteinuria. If the urine dipstick is negative, then a urine microalbumin/creatinine ratio should be obtained. 30–300 mg/g is considered microalbuminuria, and >300 mg/g is considered clinical proteinuria. In patients with proteinuria, annual creatinine measurement should be obtained.
- **Ophthalmologic monitoring:** Annual ophthalmologic evaluation should be obtained in diabetes type II patients from the time of diagnosis and diabetes type I patients 3–5 yrs after diagnosis.
- **Lipids:** Lipids should be checked q4–6mos, until goals are met. If within normal limits, patients should have yearly screening lipid panel.

- **Thyroid function:** TSH to rule out coexisting thyroid disease.
- **Foot exam:** Annually.
- **BP:** Annually.

Management

Hyperglycemia

- Complications of diabetes can be prevented or prolonged with tight blood sugar control.
- Goal HgbA1c of <7.0%, preprandial glucose of 80–120, and bedtime glucose of 100–140.
- Dietary modifications: Instruction in the proper diabetic diet is necessary. The patient does not need to completely eliminate carbohydrates but simply limit their intake. A standard American Diabetes Association diet may include 3 meals and 2–3 snacks/day. Calories should roughly be divided in the following manner: 50% carbohydrates, 30% fat, 20% protein.
- Diabetic educator: Reinforcement of ideas that you have already relayed to the patient.

Oral Agents

- **Sulfonylureas (Glipizide, Glyburide):** Stimulate pancreatic insulin secretion. Can cause significant hypoglycemia, so patients must be educated to the signs and symptoms of hypoglycemia. After dietary modifications, these have been traditional first-line agents. Traditional starting dose for glyburide is 2.5 mg PO qd, can increase to maximum of 20 mg PO qd.
- **Biguanide (Metformin):** Decreases hepatic gluconeogenesis. Does not cause hypoglycemia. Contraindicated in patients with renal/hepatic/heart failure and lactic acidosis. Medication must be discontinued 48–72 hrs before any IV contrast dye exposure and must be held for 48 hrs after such a procedure. This can be a first-line agent or can be an addition to a sulfonylurea. The usual starting dose is 500 mg PO bid; maxiumum, 2000 mg PO qd.
- **Thiazolidinediones (Rosiglitazone, Pioglitazone):** Appear to work by increasing insulin sensitivity in skeletal muscle. Contraindicated in patients with abnormal LFTs (can cause severe hepatic failure) and congestive heart failure. Monitor LFTs q2mos ×1 yr, then approximately q6mos. Should be reserved for those who have not achieved optimal blood sugar control on the above regimens.

Insulin

- Insulin is the initial therapy in patients with type I diabetes. In type II patients, insulin is usually begun when patients have been placed

TABLE 10-1.
CHARACTERISTICS OF COMMONLY USED
SUBCUTANEOUS INSULIN PREPARATIONS

Insulin	Onset	Peak (hrs)	Duration (hrs)
Lispro	5–10 mins	0.5–1	2–4
Reg	0.5–1 hr	2–4	4–6
NPH	3–4 hrs	8–14	16–24
Ultralente	4–6 hrs	10–20	24–36
Glargine	—	—	24–36

Adapted from Stoller WA. Individualizing insulin management. Three practical cases, rules for regimen adjustment. *Postgrad Med* 2002;111(5):51–66.

on the maximum dosage of metformin and a sulfonylurea and still do not have good control.

- A number of insulin formulations are available (Table 10-1):
- For 70/30 (NPH/R) formulations:
  - Begin with 0.5–1 U/kg/day.
  - Give 2/3 of dose in morning, 1/3 at night.
- For glargine formulation:
  - Start with 10 U qhs and titrate by 5–10 U until blood glucose control is achieved.
  - Can combine with oral agent or short-acting insulin.
- For short-acting lispro insulin formulation:
  - Start with 4 U before small meals, 6 U before medium meals, and 8 U before large meals.
  - Alternatively, count carbohydrates at each meal and give 1 U of mealtime lispro for every 10–15 g of carbohydrates.
- A visit to the diabetic educator for teaching in the use of insulin is essential before initiation of therapy.

Combination Therapy

Alternatives include

- Sulfonylurea + metformin
- Sulfonylurea + metformin + thiazolidinedione
- Oral agent + insulin (daytime sulfonylurea + bedtime NPH or glargine)

Cardiovascular Risk Reduction

- ASA, 81–325 mg PO qd

- Lipid reduction: Goal low-density lipoprotein is <100. Often with improved blood sugar control, dyslipidemia improves independent of a lipid-lowering agent. This is particularly true for the triglyceride levels. However, if low-density lipoprotein is not at goal, start a statin (e.g., simvastatin, 20–40 mg PO qd). Monitor LFTs (at baseline and at 6 mos).

Prevention of Renal Disease

- Monitor for microalbuminuria/proteinuria as above.

- In the presence of proteinuria/microalbuminuria, begin the patient on an ACE inhibitor or angiotensin receptor blocker (lisinopril [Zestril], 10–40 mg PO qd).

- Target BP for patients with diabetes is <130/85.

Diabetic Neuropathy

- Annual foot exam is extremely important. Foot care reduces the risk for amputation.

- Diabetic neuropathy can be extremely painful and cause diabetic patients a significant amount of distress.

- Several medications have been shown in small studies to improve the symptoms of diabetic neuropathy. These include tricyclic antidepressants, gabapentin (Neurontin), and capsaicin cream (Zostrix, Zostrix-HP). Patient response to these treatments is unpredictable and often minimal.

- Orthostatic hypotension can be treated with fludrocortisone (Florinef).

- Impotence can be treated with sildenafil (Viagra) if patients are not taking nitrates.

What to Tell the Patient

- Diabetes is a chronic illness. Lifelong control of blood glucose will reduce the risk for such complications as blindness, kidney failure, heart attack, and limb amputation.

- Blood glucose control is best achieved by taking medications and through diet and exercise.

- Close follow-up with your doctor is important to monitor for complications of diabetes.

HYPERTHYROIDISM

Etiology

See Table 10-2.

TABLE 10-2.
ETIOLOGY OF HYPERTHYROIDISM

Common	Less common	Rare
Graves' disease	Subacute thyroiditis (tender goiter)	Struma ovarii
Toxic adenoma	Postpartum thyroiditis	Hydatidiform mole
Multinodular toxic goiter	Thyrotoxicosis factitia Excess iodine ingestion with underlying thyroid disease (Jodbasedow disease)	Secondary hyperthyroidism (TSH-producing pituitary tumor; pituitary resistance to T_3 and T_4)

Key History

- **General:** Sweating, heat intolerance, weight loss, female to male ratio of 8:1 (Graves'), age (20–40).
- **HEENT:** Eye complaints (tearing, diplopia, vision loss), exophthalmos (Graves').
- **Neck:** Thyroid enlargement, nodule, neck swelling.
- **Pulmonary:** Dyspnea.
- **Cardiovascular:** Palpitations, chest pain.
- **GI:** Diarrhea, increased appetite (with possible weight gain).
- **Genitourinary:** Amenorrhea, oligomenorrhea, pregnancy (recent, current).
- **Extremities:** Leg swelling, muscle aches.
- **Neurologic:** Nervousness, fatigue, weakness, tremor.
- **Medical history:** Cardiac disease, arrhythmia (atrial fibrillation), autoimmune disorders, diabetes, myasthenia gravis, pernicious anemia.
- **Medications:** Levothyroxine (T_4), amiodarone.
- **Social history:** Immigration from iodine-deficient region (the Alps, Andes, Central Africa).
- **Family history:** Hyperthyroidism, autoimmune disorders, diabetes mellitus, myasthenia gravis, pernicious anemia.
- **In an elderly patient,** the only symptoms may be fatigue, weight loss or atrial fibrillation (apathetic hyperthyroidism).

Focused Physical Exam

- **HEENT:** Hoarse voice, diffusely enlarged (Graves' disease) vs irregular or nodular (multinodular goiter) vs tender (thyroiditis), proptosis

(Graves'), periorbital swelling (Graves'), lid lag/retraction, excess tearing, infrequent blinking

- **Neck:** Thyroid nodule/enlargement, thyroid bruit
- **Cardiovascular:** Tachycardia, irregularly irregular heart rate (atrial fibrillation), heart failure
- **Pulmonary:** Tachypnea
- **Extremities:** Pretibial myxedema (Graves'), clubbing, digital swelling (acropachy)
- **Skin:** Warm/moist/flushed, doughy skin (infiltrative dermopathy), fine hair
- **Neurologic:** Brisk reflexes, tremor

Evaluation

- **Sensitive TSH:** Initial screening test
  - Consider screening in any symptomatic patient and all women >50.
  - Decreased TSH in primary disease or factitious hyperthyroidism.
  - Elevated TSH in secondary disease.
- **Free T$_4$:** Confirmatory test if TSH <0.1µU/mL
  - Elevated free T$_4$ will confirm the diagnosis.
- **Radioactive iodine uptake scan (RAIU):** In patients with a decreased TSH and elevated free T$_4$, RAIU can help further define the diagnosis.
  - **Elevated iodine uptake:** Graves' disease (homogeneous), toxic adenoma (one hot spot), multinodular toxic goiter (multiple hot spots)
  - **Decreased iodine uptake:** Thyroiditis
- **Antithyroid antibodies** (antithyroglobulin, antithyroid peroxidase, thyroid-stimulating antibodies)
  - Likely positive in patient with Graves' disease
- **Special considerations:** Decreased TSH and normal free T$_4$
  - Likely represents euthyroid sick syndrome vs T$_3$ thyrotoxicosis.
  - Measure total T$_3$.
  - After acute setting, recheck TSH and free T$_4$ to exclude effects of severe illness on thyroid function tests.

Management

Medications

Thionamides: Propylthiouracil (PTU), 100–200 mg PO tid, methimazole (Tapazole, Thiamazole), 10–40 mg PO qd

- Medication titrated based on the T_4 level; check at 4- to 6-wk intervals until maintenance dose established.

- After 3 mos, check TSH; if elevated, indicates iatrogenic hypothyroidism, and dose should be reduced.

- Indications:

  - Conditions: Graves' disease, toxic adenoma, multinodular toxic goiter.

  - Prolonged course in patient with new diagnosis of Graves' disease in effort to achieve remission; duration of treatment 6 mos to 2 yrs (<50% likelihood long-term remission).

  - Bridge to definitive treatment (surgery or radioactive iodine [RAI] ablation).

  - Lifelong treatment in those unwilling/unable to undergo definitive treatment.

  - Thionamide treatment is ineffective in thyrotoxicosis.

- Side effects:

  - Minor: Rash, urticaria, fever, arthralgias.

  - Major: Agranulocytosis, hepatitis, vasculitis, drug-induced lupus.

  - Instruct patients to stop the drug immediately and call physician if jaundice or symptoms of agranulocytosis occur (fever, sore throat, chills).

Beta blocker therapy: Propranolol (Inderal), 20–40 mg PO qid

- Once-daily beta blockers are also effective (e.g., Atenolol).

- Beta blockade is often the sole treatment for patients with thyroiditis.

RAI:

- Indications: Graves' disease, toxic adenoma, multinodular toxic goiter.

- I^{131} ablation is safe in elderly.

- Contraindicated in children, pregnancy, lactation.

- Caution: Graves' patients with ophthalmopathy (refer to an endocrinologist).

- Side effects: hypothyroidism (15–20% at 2 yrs).

- T_4 measurements q4–6wks until T_4 stabilizes in normal range; TSH/T_4 can then be assessed q6–12mos.

Surgery

- Indications: Graves' disease (second-line therapy vs I^{131} ablation), toxic adenoma, multinodular toxic goiter.

- Caution: Graves' patients with ophthalmopathy (refer to an endocrinologist).

- Treat with a thionamide and achieve euthyroid state before surgery, then stop postop; beta blocker also administered before surgery, weaned off after surgery.

- Side effects: Hypothyroidism (5–40%), hyperthyroidism (1–3%), vocal cord paralysis, hypoparathyroidism.

- T_4 measurements q4–6wks until T_4 stabilizes in normal range; TSH/T_4 can then be assessed q6–12mos.

Difficult Management Situations

Subclinical Hyperthyroidism

- Currently, no good guidelines for treatment.

- Patients at risk for osteoporosis and atrial fibrillation.

- Consider treating patients if
  - symptomatic
  - elderly
  - underlying cardiac disease

- Consider referring these patients to an endocrinologist for a second opinion.

Thyrotoxic Crisis (Thyroid Storm)

- Patients with hyperthyroidism who undergo surgery, are given radiocontrast, or are under severe stress are at risk.

- Signs and symptoms: Hyperpyrexia, flushing, marked tachycardia/atrial fibrillation, cardiac failure.

- Need to be hospitalized under care of an endocrinologist.

When to Refer

Refer to an endocrinologist for

- secondary hyperthyroidism

- goiters or nodules
- pediatric/adolescent patients
- pregnancy/postpartum
- difficult management situations (ischemic heart disease, patients on lithium or amiodarone)
- subclinical hyperthyroidism

Refer to a dermatologist for significant skin findings, and refer to an ophthalmologist for eye complaints.

What to Tell the Patient

- Treatment of hyperthyroidism may result in side effects, which can be serious; therefore, close follow-up during treatment is essential.
- Side effect of I^{131} ablation and thyroidectomy is risk of hypothyroidism and may require thyroid replacement.
- Untreated/undertreated hyperthyroidism can have serious sequelae: atrial fibrillation, osteoporosis, heart failure, and even thyroid storm.

HYPOTHYROIDISM

Etiology

See Table 10-3.

Key History

- **General:** gender (female), fatigue, cold intolerance, weight gain

TABLE 10-3.
ETIOLOGY OF HYPOTHYROIDISM

Primary hypothyroidism: "gland failure" (99%)	Secondary hypothyroidism: "hypothalamic-pituitary axis failure" (1%)
Autoimmune: Hashimoto's thyroiditis	**Hypothalamic dysfunction:** neoplasm, TB, sarcoid, radiation exposure
Iatrogenic: I^{131} ablation, thyroidectomy	**Pituitary dysfunction:** Neoplasm, surgery, idiopathic, Sheehan's syndrome, Cushing's syndrome, radiation exposure
Drug induced: Iodine deficiency/excess, lithium, amiodarone, antithyroid drugs	
Congenital: Thyroid agenesis/dysgenesis, biosynthetic defect	

- **HEENT:** hair loss, hoarseness, decreased hearing, taste, smell
- **GI:** constipation
- **Genitourinary:** menstrual irregularities (amenorrhea, menorrhagia)
- **Orthopedic:** arthralgias, myalgias
- **Neurologic:** headaches
- **Medical history:** autoimmune diseases (Addison's, primary biliary cirrhosis, diabetes mellitus type I), hypercholesterolemia
- **Medications:** lithium, amiodarone, iodine, interferon alpha
- **Social history:** immigration from iodine-deficient region (the Alps, Andes, Central Africa)
- **Family history:** hypothyroidism

Focused Physical Exam

- **General:** lethargic appearance, pallor, slow reaction time, hoarse voice
- **HEENT:** coarse thin hair, thin lateral eyebrows, periorbital edema, hearing loss
- **Neck:** goiter
- **Cardiovascular:** bradycardia, distant heart sounds (pericardial effusion)
- **Breast:** galactorrhea
- **Pulmonary:** slow respiratory rate, decreased breath sounds/dullness to percussion at bases (pleural effusion)
- **Extremities:** peripheral nonpitting edema, brittle nails
- **Skin:** orange hue, dry/coarse/cold skin, poor turgor
- **Neurologic:** delayed relaxation phase of reflexes

Evaluation

- **Sensitive TSH:**
  - Screening test for hypothyroidism.
  - Consider screening in any symptomatic patient and all women >50.
  - Elevated TSH in primary disease.
  - Decreased TSH in secondary disease.
- **Free T_4:** Confirmatory test for hypothyroidism.

- **Antithyroid antibodies:** If positive, indicates autoimmune disease.

- **CBC:** Normocytic or macrocytic anemia.

- **Cholesterol:** Often elevated.

- **Prolactin:** May be elevated.

- **Chemistries:** Decreased Na^+ and glucose, elevated LFTs and creatine kinase.

- **MRI head:** Consider in evaluation for pituitary tumor.

- **Special considerations:** Decreased TSH and normal free T_4. Likely indicates subclinical hypothyroidism, or amiodarone effect.

Management

- In treating primary hypothyroidism, goal is to replace thyroid hormone until TSH is in euthyroid range.

- **Levothyroxine (Synthroid):**

  - Young patient without cardiac history: Start with 50–75 µg PO qd; increase by 25 µg q6–8wks (until TSH in euthyroid range).

  - Elderly patients and patients with heart disease: Start with 25–50 µg PO qd; increase by 25 µg q6–8wks (until TSH in euthyroid range).

- **Labs to follow during therapy:**

  - **Primary hypothyroidism:** Recheck TSH 6–8 wks after initiation of levothyroxine and 6–8 wks after each dose change; once stable, check q yr.

  - **Secondary hypothyroidism:** Follow free T_4.

- If TSH is still elevated after levothyroxine has been initiated, consider the following before increasing dose:

  - Is the patient actually taking the medication?

  - Could any other substances be interfering with absorption (e.g., aluminum antacids, calcium or iron supplements, sucralfate, cholestyramine)?

Difficult Management Situations
- **Subclinical hypothyroidism:**

  - Currently no good treatment guidelines

  - Consider treatment if

- symptomatic
- elderly females
- antithyroid antibodies present: 5%/yr risk of converting to overt hypothyroidism
- high TSH (>10): The higher the TSH, the more likely to convert to overt hypothyroidism
- hyperlipidemia present

When to Refer

Refer to endocrinologist for

- secondary hypothyroidism
- poorly controlled patients (despite appropriate dose adjustments)
- patients with goiters or nodules

What to Tell the Patient

- The medication for hypothyroidism is the same as the hormone naturally produced by their bodies.
- Their bodies have an intrinsic signaling mechanism that indicates how much hormone is needed; because every person is different, the correct dose will be determined with lab testing.
- Because the medication must be adjusted, close physician follow-up is essential.
- *The medication takes 4–6 wks to work*; patients will not feel better overnight, but rather over the next few weeks.
- Not taking the medication and taking excess doses of the medication can have serious side effects.

SOLITARY THYROID NODULE

A palpable discrete swelling within an otherwise normal-appearing gland.

Characteristics of Thyroid Nodules

Benign solitary nodule	Thyroid cancer
Increased age	Extremes of age (very old or young)
Female gender	Male gender
External radiation	External radiation
	Family history of papillary, medullary carcinoma; multiple endocrine neoplasia II syndrome; familial polyposis (Gardner's syndrome)

Differential Diagnosis

- Benign nodule
- Colloid (adenomatous) nodule
- Follicular adenomas
- Malignant nodules
- Carcinoma (papillary, follicular, medullary, anaplastic)
- Thyroid cysts

Key History

- **General:** age (young increases cancer risk), gender (male increases cancer risk), weight loss
- **Neck:** lymph node enlargement, voice changes (vocal cord paralysis)
- **Thyroid:** rate of nodule growth, symptoms of hyperthyroidism, lymphadenopathy
- **Medical history:** other benign thyroid illness, pancreatic/parathyroid tumors (MEN II)
- **Family history:** papillary or medullary carcinoma, MEN II syndrome, familial adenomatous polyposis
- **Social history:** radiation exposure

Focused Physical Exam

- **Any signs of hyper- or hypothyroidism** (see Hyperthyroidism and Hypothyroidism)
- **Neck:**
  - goiter (palpate thyroid from behind as patient swallows water)
  - nodule size (needs to be >1 cm to be palpable)
  - nodule location
  - nodule texture (multiple, smooth, soft, mobile nodule suggests benign; hard, fixed nodule with associated lymphadenopathy suggests cancer)
  - thyroid bruit
- **Lymph:** peripheral lymphadenopathy

Evaluation

Thyroid Function Tests

- **TSH:** Screen for thyrotoxicosis or hypothyroidism.

- **Free T$_4$:** Confirmatory test if TSH abnormal.
- **Serum thyroglobulin:**
  - Elevated in metastatic follicular/papillary carcinoma.
  - Follow to assess for cancer recurrence.
  - Falsely elevated in thyroiditis.

Calcitonin

Elevated in medullary carcinoma but nonspecific (also elevated in thyroiditis, hypercalcemia, pregnancy, azotemia, other malignancies).

Fine-Needle Aspiration (FNA)

Initial test recommended for evaluation of a solitary thyroid nodule (false-negative rate <5%). Cytologic results:

- **Benign:** can safely follow clinically (70%)
- **Malignant:** oncology referral and intervention based on cancer type (5%)
- **Indeterminate:** mandates further testing to rule out carcinoma (15%)
- **Follicular cells:** referral to surgery (cannot distinguish benign vs malignant follicular cells on FNA)

Thyroiditis with a Thyroid Nodule

Thyroiditis can coexist with a thyroid nodule: *Do not let this deter pursuit of diagnostic evaluation.*

Radionuclide Scanning

- Less commonly used with widespread needle biopsy availability.
- In patients with an indeterminate nodule, a "hot" or hyperfunctioning nodule is usually benign.
- Solitary nodules in patient with hyperthyroidism: useful in differentiating toxic adenoma vs Graves' disease.

U/S

- Uses: Identifies cystic lesions, provides follow-up of a lesion size, helps direct FNA.
- Preferred imaging technique over CT or MRI.

Management

Malignant Lesions

- Surgery based on tumor type.

- Lifelong thyroxine therapy (suppresses TSH).

Indeterminate Lesions

Surgery for all patients vs short-term thyroxine therapy (if the nodule is present after thyroxine, surgery is absolutely indicated).

Cystic Lesions

- >50% disappear with aspiration.

- If aspiration is bloody or nodule recurs, consider surgical removal.

Benign Nodules

Observation with repeated clinical evaluation.

Thyroxine Therapy

- Growth during thyroxine suppression is an indication for surgery.

- Goal: suppress the TSH to 0.2–0.4 µU/mL for 6 mos, during which time one should follow nodule size and thyroglobulin levels.

- If the nodule decreases, extend treatment to keep the TSH within the low to normal range (<15% of benign nodules respond to this treatment).

- Used in limited cases (weigh benefit vs side effects, such as osteoporosis, atrial fibrillation, worsen cardiac disease).

When to Refer

Refer all patients with indeterminate or malignant FNAs to an endocrinologist or surgeon.

What to Tell the Patient

- The majority of solitary thyroid nodules are benign but warrant evaluation to detect potential malignancies in their early stages.

- Thyroid cancer can be often effectively treated and even curable with early detection.

OSTEOPOROSIS

A deterioration of bone tissue resulting in decreased bone mass density and increased bone fragility.

Classification

Primary vs Secondary

- **Primary:** Decrease in bone mass density unrelated to other underlying illness (function of aging and decreased gonadal function).

- **Secondary:** Related to chronic medical conditions, genetic disorders, medications, and nutritional states that predispose one to decreased bone mass.

Type I vs Type II

- **Type I "postmenopausal osteoporosis":** Trabecular bone loss (vertebral) in postmenopausal women.

- **Type II "senile osteoporosis":** Cortical bone loss (femur, pelvis), in both genders, particularly >70 yrs.

Risk Factors

- Female gender

- Older age

- Race (whites, Asians > African-Americans, Hispanics)

- Hormone deficiency

- Early menopause

- Poor nutrition

- Low physical activity/immobility

- Alcohol/tobacco abuse, high caffeine intake

- Medications (corticosteroids, heparin, aluminum-containing antacids)

- Medical conditions (Cushing's, thyrotoxicosis, liver disease, renal disease)

- Genetic disorders (Marfan's, osteogenesis imperfecta)

Key History

- **General:** weight loss

- **Back:** upper or midthoracic back pain (from compression fractures; increases with sitting, decreases with rest)

- **Medications:** corticosteroids, heparin, aluminum-containing antacids (dosage, duration)

- **Medical history:** Cushing's, thyrotoxicosis, hyperparathyroidism, liver disease, renal disease, genetic disorders (e.g., Marfan's), age of menopause, previous fracture (especially distal radius and hip)

- **Social history:** diet (caffeine, alcohol, and tobacco), activity level, history of falls

- **Family history:** osteoporosis

Focused Physical Exam

- **General:** cachexia (consider dietary screen, cancer evaluation)

- **HEENT:** lid lag, goiter (hyperthyroidism); moon facies, buffalo hump (Cushing's)

- **Skin:** thin, fragile

- **Orthopedic:** hip or distal arm deformity (previous fracture)

- **Back:** vertebral tenderness (compression fracture), Dowager's hump, loss of height

Evaluation

Dual-Energy X-Ray Absorptiometry (DEXA)

- **T score:** Number of standard deviations above or below the mean bone density vs young controls

- **Z score:** Number of standard deviations above or below the mean bone density vs age-matched controls

- **WHO guidelines for diagnosis of osteoporosis (by T score):** see Table 10-4.

- **DEXA is recommended** in the following patients:

  - perimenopausal women (willing to undergo treatment for osteoporosis)

  - any postmenopausal woman with a fracture

  - all women >65

  - postmenopausal women <65 with 1 or more risk factors for osteoporosis

  - those with radiographic evidence of decreased bone density

  - patients on long-term glucocorticoid therapy

TABLE 10-4.
WHO GUIDELINES
FOR OSTEOPOROSIS DIAGNOSIS

T score	Diagnosis
> -1	Normal
-1 to -2.5	Osteopenia
< -2.5	Osteoporosis
< -2.5 with fracture	Severe osteoporosis

- those with asymptomatic hyperparathyroidism

- when monitoring therapeutic effect in patient on therapy for osteoporosis

Lab Testing

No specific lab abnormalities are associated with osteoporosis (useful primarily in ruling out secondary causes of osteoporosis).

- **Chemistries:** Creatinine (renal failure), liver functions (hepatic disease), phosphorus and calcium (osteomalacia, hyperparathyroidism), alkaline phosphatase (Paget's, fracture, liver disease).

- **TSH:** Hyperthyroidism.

- **CBC:** Anemia, multiple myeloma.

- **Serum protein electrophoresis/urine protein electrophoresis:** Multiple myeloma.

- **Sex hormones:** Estrogen, testosterone, luteinizing hormone and follicle-stimulating hormone (hypogonadism).

- **25-Hydroxy-vitamin D level:** Osteomalacia.

- **Dexamethasone suppression test, 24-hr urine cortisol:** Cushing's.

- **X-rays:** Consider plain films of the spine to rule out compression fractures in any patient with vertebral tenderness on exam.

Management

When to Initiate Therapy

- All postmenopausal women with fracture of the radius, hip, vertebra

- T score <2.5 standard deviations below the mean, and <1.5 below mean in those with additional risk factors

Behavior Modification

- Avoid tobacco, alcohol, caffeine use.

- Eat a balanced diet.

- Exercise regularly (30–60 mins 3×/wk).

Nutritional Therapy

- **Elemental calcium (calcium carbonate)** 1500 mg PO qd: recommended in women >50 on hormone replacement therapy and anyone >65

- **Vitamin D** 400–1000 IU PO qd

- Physiologic replacement, shown to decrease rate of nonvertebral fractures in the elderly

- Aids in increasing intestinal calcium absorption

Pharmacologic Treatment

- **Hormone replacement therapy** (see Chap. 23, Women's Health)

- **Calcitonin,** 200 IU intranasally qd or 50–100 IU SQ/IM qd

  - Inhibits bone reabsorption and decreases bone pain.

  - Often prescribed for acute osteoporotic fracture.

  - The increase in bone density achieved from calcitonin may be transient and overall significantly less than that achieved with estrogen or bisphosphonates.

- **Bisphosphonates:** Alendronate, 5 mg PO qd or 35 mg PO q wk (prevention dose) or 10 mg PO qd or 70 mg PO q wk (osteoporosis dose)

  - Binds to mineralized bone and inhibits osteoclast activity.

  - Consider in osteoporosis secondary to estrogen deficiency, immobilization, and glucocorticoid treatment.

  - Continuous high doses can result in impaired bone mineralization.

  - Side effects: esophagitis, gastritis.

  - Patient must take on empty stomach, drink 8 oz H_2O, and stay upright for 30 mins after dose to minimize risk of esophagitis.

- **Selective estrogen receptor modulators:** Raloxifene, 60 mg PO qd

  - Side effects: hot flashes, elevated risk of deep venous thrombosis and pulmonary embolism.

When to Refer

Refer to endocrinologist for patients with secondary causes of osteoporosis.

Difficult Management Situations

Patients taking glucocorticoids are at high risk for osteoporosis.

- Use lowest dose possible of steroids.

- Regular weight-bearing exercise.

- Calcium and vitamin D supplements.

- Administer estrogen or bisphosphonate. If bone mineral density is still low with single agent, consider combination therapy (estrogen and bisphosphonate). Measure bone mineral density q6–12mos for the first 2 yrs of treatment to assess efficacy of therapy.

What to Tell the Patient

- Explain the risk factors for osteoporosis and encourage modification to degree possible (recommend regular weight-bearing exercise and advise tobacco, alcohol, and caffeine cessation).

- Osteoporosis is a silent disorder without signs or symptoms until late-stage consequences; therefore, early diagnosis and intervention are necessary.

SUGGESTED READING

Clinical Guidelines Part 2: Screening for thyroid disease: an update. *Ann Intern Med* 1998;129:144–158.

Cooper DS. Subclinical hypothyroidism. *N Engl J Med* 2001;345:512–516.

Eastell R. Treatment of postmenopausal osteoporosis. *N Engl J Med* 1998;338:736–746.

Hermus AR, Huysmans DA. Treatment of benign nodular thyroid disease. *N Engl J Med* 1998; 338:1438–1447.

Mazzaferri, EL. Management of a solitary thyroid nodule. *N Engl J Med* 1993;328:553–559.

The National Institutes of Health (NIH)–sponsored *Consensus Development Conference on Osteoporosis Prevention, Diagnosis, and Therapy*. Bethesda, MD: March 27–29, 2000.

South-Paul JE. Osteoporosis: part I. Evaluation and assessment. *Am Fam Physician* 2001;63:897–904.

South-Paul JE. Osteoporosis: part II. Pharmacologic and nonpharmacologic treatment. *Am Fam Physician* 2001;63:1121–1128.

Stoller WA. Individualizing insulin management: three practical cases, rules for regimen adjustment. *Postgrad Med* 2002;111(5):51–66.

Toft AD. Subclinical hypothyroidism. *N Engl J Med* 2001;345:512–516.

Vanderpump MP, Ahlquist JA, et al. Consensus statement for good practice and audit measures in the management of hypothyroidism and hyperthyroidism. *BMJ* 1996;313:539–544.

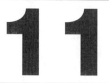

Ear, Nose, and Throat Diseases

I've had it up to my ears . . .

ALLERGIC RHINITIS

Definition

Allergic rhinitis is caused by hypersensitivity to inhaled allergens, causing symptoms such as congestion, rhinorrhea, and sneezing.

Differential Diagnosis

- Acute infections (viral or bacterial)
- Rhinitis medicamentosa
- Vasomotor rhinitis
- Nasal septal obstruction

Key History

- **General:** duration of symptoms, seasonal variation, triggers (e.g., pets, grass, pollen), age of onset (usually <20)
- **HEENT:** congestion, rhinorrhea, watery eyes, sneezing, fever, purulent nasal drainage, headache
- **Pulmonary:** dyspnea
- **Medical history:** asthma, eczema, urticaria
- **Medications:** previous medications used (including over the counter), ASA, NSAIDs, ACE inhibitors, beta blockers
- **Family history:** asthma, eczema, urticaria
- **Social history:** inhaled drug use (cocaine), work exposures, home environment (carpeting, pets, dust), smoking

Focused Physical Exam

- **HEENT:** boggy nasal mucosa, nasal polyps, deviated septum, nasal septal perforation, ocular injection, "allergic shiners"
- **Pulmonary:** wheezes (asthma)
- **Skin:** eczema, rash, urticaria

Evaluation

Generally, very little workup is required besides a good history and physical exam. Consider allergy skin testing for potential allergens.

Management

Environmental Controls

- Use dust encasings (for pillow and mattress), remove carpeting, remove pets (at least from bedroom), close windows, and use air conditioning during pollen season.

- Avoid allergens as much as possible.

Oral Antihistamines

First Generation

- Diphenhydramine (Benadryl), 25–50 mg PO q4–6h or qhs.

- Available over the counter. Major side effects include sedation and anticholinergic reactions (urinary retention, dry mouth), particularly in elderly patients.

Second Generation

- Cetirizine (Zyrtec), 10 mg PO qd; fexofenadine (Allegra), 180 mg PO qd or 60 mg PO bid; loratadine (Claritin), 10 mg PO qd.

- Loratadine is available over the counter; cetirizine and fexofenadine are available by prescription only.

- Second-generation antihistamines have much less sedative effects and fewer drug interactions.

Nasal Sprays

Nasal Steroids

- Budesonide (Rhinocort), 2 sprays/nostril bid; fluticasone (Flonase), 2 sprays/nostril qd; mometasone (Nasonex), 2 sprays/nostril qd.

- Danger of septal perforation with prolonged use; monitor via regular nasal exam.

Nonsteroid Nasal Sprays

- Azelastine (Astelin), 2 sprays/nostril bid.

- Caution with oxymetazoline (Afrin); limit use to <3 days to avoid rebound congestion.

Ocular Decongestants

- Useful for patients with eye symptoms.

- Naphcon-A, 1–2 gtts bid–qid prn (over the counter)

- Olopatadine (Patanol), 1–2 gtts OU bid

Immunotherapy

- Immunotherapy is an option for long-term control if the patient has positive skin tests.

Antibiotics

- Antibiotics are not indicated unless there is evidence of bacterial infection (fever, purulent nasal drainage).

When to Refer

- Refer to an allergist if symptoms are difficult to control and/or if considering skin testing or immunotherapy.
- Refer to an otolaryngologist if anatomic abnormalities are suspected.

What to Tell the Patient

- Maintaining an allergen-free environment is extremely important for symptom control.

OTITIS MEDIA

Definition

Infection of the middle ear. Occurs most commonly in children but can occur in adults as well.

Etiology

- Bacterial (*Streptococcus pneumoniae*, *Haemophilus influenzae*, *Moraxella catarrhalis*, Group A *Streptococcus*, *Pseudomonas aeruginosa*)
- Serous (upper respiratory infection, allergic rhinitis, cerebrospinal fluid leak, hemotympanum)
- Mechanical obstruction (cholesteatoma, eustachian tube dysfunction)

Differential Diagnosis

- Acute otitis externa
- Mastoiditis
- Carcinoma
- Cerebrospinal fluid leak
- Hemotympanum

Key History

General: fever

HEENT: ear pain, hearing loss (characteristic of bacterial infection); discharge, pressure, fullness, popping, hearing loss (characteristic of serous infection)

Medical history: sinusitis, allergic rhinitis, eustachian tube dysfunction, trauma

Focused Physical Exam

- **Vital signs:** BP, heart rate, temperature.
- **HEENT:**
  - Tympanic membrane hyperemia, opacification, loss of landmarks
  - Mastoid tenderness, postauricular swelling, and erythema (suggests mastoiditis)
  - Amber-colored fluid (suggests serous OM), decreased mobility with pneumatic otoscopy
- **Red flag:** Unilateral serous OM in an adult rarely is associated with nasopharyngeal cancer.

Evaluation

Diagnosis is generally made from history and physical exam.

Management

Acute Bacterial Otitis Media

- Amoxicillin (Amoxil), 500 mg PO qid ×10 days, or cefuroxime (Ceftin), 500 mg PO bid ×10 days.
- TMP-SMX (Bactrim, Septra), 1 tablet PO bid ×10 days, or azithromycin (Zithromax), 500 mg PO × 1, then 250 mg PO qd × 4 days for penicillin-allergic patients.

Otitis Media with Effusion

- Effusion can last up to several weeks after resolution of acute OM.
- Should be followed until resolution; does not need treatment if no evidence of reinfection or hearing loss.

Serous Otitis Media

A combination antihistamine/decongestant can be helpful for symptomatic relief.

Surgical Treatment

Surgery is indicated for recurrent, symptomatic infections and for removal of tumors or cholesteatomas. Surgical options include myringotomy tubes for selected patients.

When to Refer

Refer to an otolaryngologist in cases of OM with effusion or recurrent OM that may require myringotomy or if removal of cholesteatoma or other tumor is necessary.

What to Tell the Patient

- OM can progress to such complications as mastoiditis, brain abscess, and meningitis if incompletely treated.

- Recurrent OM may require placement of ear tubes for drainage.

OTITIS EXTERNA

Definition

Infection of the external auditory canal (EAC). Two stages of infection:

- Acute stage, typified by pain and swelling in the EAC.
- Chronic stage, characterized by thickening of the EAC skin, dry and flaky EAC skin, and canal narrowing.

Etiology

- *Pseudomonas aeruginosa*
- *Staphylococcus aureus*
- Fungal organisms

Differential Diagnosis

- Malignant otitis externa (fulminant EAC infection)
- Perichondritis/chondritis
- Furunculosis
- Contact dermatitis
- Otomycosis
- Cellulitis

Key History

- **HEENT:** pain with movement of helix or tragus, pruritus, hearing loss, "plugging" sensation

- **Risk factors:** increased heat and humidity, allergies, trauma, swimming

- **Medical history:** diabetes (increased risk of malignant otitis externa), HIV, chronic illnesses (more likely to have fungal infections), immunosuppression

Red Flags for Otitis Externa

Presence of a red flag warrants evaluation by an otolaryngologist!

- Inflammation and swelling of the pinna → perichondritis/chondritis

- Ear discharge → malignant otitis externa

- Deep, boring pain → malignant otitis externa

- Cranial nerve deficits → Ramsay Hunt syndrome (herpes zoster oticus), malignant otitis externa

- Herpetic lesions → Ramsay Hunt syndrome

Focused Physical Exam

- **Vital signs:** fever

- **HEENT:** swelling of pinna, ear discharge, herpetic lesions, rash

- **Neurologic:** cranial nerve deficits

Evaluation

History and physical exam usually make diagnosis; beware of red flags.

Management

- **Keep EAC clean and dry.** Patient should use silicon ear plugs or petroleum jelly–soaked cotton balls in the ears during showers.

- **Antibiotic eardrops:**

  - Hydrocortisone/polymyxin/neomycin otic, 4 gtts in ear ×7–10 days

  - Ciprofloxacin otic, 0.3% 1 gtt bid ×7–10 days

- **Decrease recurrence** by drying the EAC with alcohol drops after swimming, then applying antibiotic drops or a 2% acetic acid solution.

  - Swim-Ear (isopropyl alcohol/anhydrous glycerins) for drying

  - Home remedy: 1/3 white vinegar, 2/3 rubbing alcohol for drying

When to Refer

Refer to an otolaryngologist for any red flag symptoms or persistent infections.

What to Tell the Patient

- Otitis externa is an infection of the outer ear canal.

- No swimming or submersion of head while the infection is being treated.

- Prevent recurrences by drying the ear thoroughly after swimming.

CERUMEN IMPACTION

Key History

- **HEENT:** Conductive hearing loss, "full" sensation, tinnitus, dizziness, ear discomfort

- **Medical history:** Use of cotton swabs to clean ears

Focused Physical Exam

- **HEENT:** Copious amounts of cerumen blocking canal, foreign body, bloody or malodorous discharge (indicates perforated tympanic membrane)

Evaluation

History and physical exam to rule out foreign body, otitis media, and perforated tympanic membrane

Management

- Do not remove cerumen if symptoms of a perforated tympanic membrane are present!

- To perform a **cerumenectomy:**

  - Have the patient instill neomycin sulfate (Cortisporin) eardrops or mineral oil bid–tid ×1 wk.

  - Irrigate the canal with warm water using a large-bore irrigation tip (e.g., 10- or 20-cc syringe).

  - Repeat as needed. Consider breaking up the wax with a curette if necessary.

  - Dry the canal with cotton swabs.

- **Alternative treatment:** Over-the-counter wax softeners, such as triethanolamine. Instill the drops as needed for 15–30 mins each time until wax is softened and cleared.

When to Refer

Refer to an otolaryngologist for a perforated tympanic membrane.

What to Tell the Patient

- Cerumen or "ear wax" is produced by your body and generally clears on its own.

- Do not use cotton tips to clean your ears; they will push the cerumen further into the canal.

- Prevent recurrences by using over-the-counter wax softeners.

HEARING LOSS

Definition

Conductive Hearing Loss

- Usually a defect in the external or middle ear that impairs passage of sound to the cochlea.

- Common causes: cerumen impaction, fluid, tumors, trauma, otosclerosis.

Sensorineural Hearing Loss

- Caused by damage to cranial nerve VIII.

- Etiologies: ototoxic medications, Ménière's disease, trauma, noise-induced hearing loss, MS, autoimmune diseases, presbycusis, tumors (acoustic neuroma).

Mixed

- Both conductive and sensorineural hearing loss.

- May be caused by trauma, otosclerosis, or chronic otitis media.

Key History

- **Symptoms:** difficulty hearing, dementia-like symptoms, social withdrawal/isolation, vertigo, tinnitus (Ménière's disease)

- **Medical history:** recent upper respiratory infection, MS, autoimmune diseases

- **Medications:** current and past medications (aminoglycosides, loop diuretics, vancomycin, cisplatin)

- **Social history:** exposure to noise, occupational history

Focused Physical Exam

- **HEENT:** cerumen, signs of infection, tympanic membrane scarring/perforation, fluid in middle ear canal.

- **Neurologic:** cranial nerve deficits.

- **Weber test:** Place a vibrating tuning fork in center of patient's forehead or on the bridge of the nose. Ask the patient on which side noise is heard. Detects both conductive and sensorineural hearing loss.

  - If patient hears noise in **both** ears, the patient has normal hearing **or** bilateral hearing loss.

  - If sound is louder on the **right,** patient has right-sided conductive hearing loss **or** left-sided sensorineural hearing loss.

  - If sound is louder on the **left,** patient has left-sided conductive hearing loss **or** right-sided sensorineural hearing loss.

- **Rinné test:** Place a vibrating tuning fork on the patient's mastoid bone, then move to 2 cm away from the external auditory canal. Ask the patient to tell you in which position the sound is louder. Detects conductive hearing loss.

  - If **air conduction is better** than bone conduction, patient has no conductive hearing loss.

  - If **bone conduction is better** than air conduction, patient has conductive hearing loss.

Evaluation

- Audiometric testing is useful in all patients with hearing loss to delineate severity and to document need for hearing aids.

- In a patient with fluid in the middle ear canal without a history of previous trauma or upper respiratory infection (especially if fluid is unilateral), evaluation for a tumor is necessary!

Management

Treatment is based on the underlying cause:

- Cerumen impaction: See Cerumen Impaction.

- Otitis media: See Otitis Media.

Hearing aids are beneficial when indicated (based on audiometric testing).

When to Refer

- Refer to an audiologist for audiometric testing.

- Refer to an otolaryngologist for evaluation of suspected tumor or for cases in which the diagnosis is unclear.

What to Tell the Patient

- Hearing loss is a common result of aging (presbycusis). However, all hearing loss should be evaluated to rule out other causes.

- Sudden hearing loss should be evaluated immediately.

- Avoid sustained exposure to loud noises, or use earplugs if exposure is necessary.

- Hearing aids can greatly improve quality of life.

PHARYNGITIS

Etiology

- **Bacterial:** Group A *Streptococcus*, Group C *Streptococcus*, *N. gonorrhea*, *Arcanobacterium haemolyticum*

- **Viral:** Rhinovirus, adenovirus, influenza, herpes simplex virus, Epstein-Barr virus, coronavirus

- **Other:** Postnasal drip (sinusitis or allergic rhinitis), candidiasis, GERD (laryngeal reflux)

Key History

- **General:** onset, duration of symptoms, fever, sick contacts

- **HEENT:** pain with swallowing, postnasal drainage, cough, rhinorrhea

- **GI:** abdominal pain, nausea, vomiting

- **Medical history:** rheumatic fever or poststreptococcal glomerulonephritis

- **Social history:** orogenital sexual activity, sexual abuse

Focused Physical Exam

- **Vital signs:** fever

- **HEENT:** rhinorrhea, pharyngeal erythema, pharyngeal exudate, enlarged tonsils, anterior cervical lymphadenopathy (*Strep* infection); anterior and posterior cervical lymphadenopathy (Epstein-Barr virus)

- **Cardiovascular:** murmurs

- **Abdominal:** hepatosplenomegaly (Epstein-Barr virus)

- **Skin:** Scarlatiniform rash

Evaluation

See Fig. 11-1.

Management

- **Symptomatic management:** fluids, salt water gargles, over-the-counter lozenges, and analgesics, especially for viral pharyngitis.

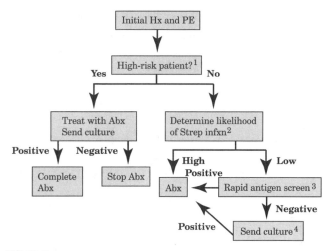

FIG. 11-1.
Algorithm for pharyngitis evaluation. [1]High-risk patients: history of rheumatic fever, valvular disease, or poststrep glomerulonephritis, or household member with same history. [2]Suggestive: <3 days of fever >39°C, tender anterior cervical lymph nodes, enlarged tonsils with purulent exudates. [3]Rapid antigen screen is 60–90% sensitive and 85–99% specific. [4]Culture is 99% sensitive. Consider culture for *Neisseria gonorrhea* if indicated. Consider candidiasis in immunocompromised patient. Abx, antibiotics; Hx, history; infxn, infection; PE, physical exam.

- **Group A streptococcal infection:**
  - Penicillin VK, 500 mg PO bid ×10 days, or benzathine penicillin G, 1.2 million U IM ×1.
  - If penicillin allergic: erythromycin, 250 mg PO qid or 500 mg PO bid ×10 days.

- ***N. gonorrhea* infection:**
  - Ceftriaxone, 125 mg IM ×1. Consider also treating empirically with doxycycline, 100 mg PD bid ×7 days, to cover chlamydial infections, as these two often co-exist.
  - Consider pelvic exam/cervical cultures for gonorrhea/chlamydia for women and urethral cultures for men.
  - Advise patient to notify sexual partners.

- **Epstein-Barr virus:**
  - Symptomatic treatment.

- Advise patient to avoid contact sports until splenomegaly resolves (due to risk of splenic rupture).
- **Oral candidiasis:** Nystatin swish and swallow, 4–6 mg PO qid.
- **GERD:**
  - Proton-pump inhibitors are the most effective treatment for laryngeal reflux; H$_2$-blockers are ineffective.
  - See Chap. 13, Gastroenterology, for more therapeutic options.

When to Refer

Refer to an otolaryngologist or to the ED immediately for drainage for suspected retropharyngeal or peritonsillar abscess.

What to Tell the Patient

- Most sore throats are caused by viral infections, which do not require antibiotic therapy.
- If you have a bacterial infection, take antibiotics for the full course, even if you start to feel better.
- Rare but serious complications of untreated *Strep* throat include acute rheumatic fever and acute renal failure from poststreptococcal glomerulonephritis.
- Return to your physician if you have persistent fever, increased difficulty swallowing, or hematuria.

SINUSITIS

Etiology

- **Bacterial:**
  - Acute: *Streptococcus pneumoniae, Haemophilus influenzae, M. catarrhalis,* group A beta-hemolytic *Streptococcus*
  - Chronic: anaerobes, *Corynebacterium, S. aureus*
- **Viral**
- **Fungal:** Mucor, aspergillus
- **Mechanical obstruction:** Polyps, tumor, deviated septum

Key History

- **General:** duration of symptoms (acute <3 wks, subacute >3 wks and <3 mos, chronic >3 mos), fever, failure for recent upper respiratory infection to resolve
- **Head:** frontal headache, sinus pain that worsens with leaning forward, retroorbital pain

- **Ear:** earache
- **Nose:** postnasal drip, nasal congestion, chronic cough, purulent/ green nasal discharge
- **Oropharynx:** sore throat, maxillary tooth pain
- **Medical history/risk factors:**
  - **For bacterial infection:** allergic rhinitis, upper respiratory infection, deviated septum, nasal polyps, cigarette smoke, dental extraction, barotrauma, foreign body, uncontrolled diabetes mellitus
  - **For fungal infection:** radiation therapy, immunosuppression, long-term antibiotic or steroid use
  - **Other:** hypogammaglobulinemia, cystic fibrosis, immotile cilia syndrome, bronchiectasis, allergic bronchopulmonary aspergillosis (sinusitis, asthma, nasal polyps)
  - **Medications:** antibiotics, nasal decongestants, antihistamines, ACE inhibitors, beta blockers, NSAIDs, ASA

Focused Physical Exam

- **Vital signs:** fever
- **Head:** sinus tenderness with palpation/percussion, decreased transillumination
- **Eyes:** pain with eye movement, dilated pupils (cavernous sinus thrombosis); impaired extraocular movement, ptosis, proptosis, diplopia (orbital cellulitis)
- **Nose:** hyperemia, purulent discharge, nasal polyps, septal deviation, foreign bodies
- **Oropharynx:** fetid breath (chronic sinusitis)
- **Neurologic:** cranial nerve deficits, meningeal signs

Red Flags for Complications of Sinusitis

- Pain with eye movement, ptosis, proptosis → orbital cellulitis
- Impaired extraocular movement, dilated pupil → cavernous sinus thrombosis
- Fever, stiff neck, mental status changes → meningitis, brain abscess
- Bone pain, persistent fever → osteomyelitis
- Wheezing, evidence of bronchospasm → asthma
- Chronic infection not responding to treatment → fungal sinusitis
- Black, necrotic turbinates → mucormycosis

Evaluation

- **Diagnosis is generally made clinically.**

- **Limited CT of sinuses** is indicated if the patient has chronic sinusitis or is not responding to therapy, or if mechanical obstruction is suspected as the cause.

- **Biopsy** is usually needed for definitive diagnosis of fungal sinusitis.

Management

Acute bacterial sinusitis resolves on its own much of the time. Antibiotics should be used judiciously due to risks of side effects and increasing resistance. However, studies have shown that antibiotics may shorten the course of infection and result in higher cure rates.

- **Antibiotic therapy:**

  - Amoxicillin, 500 mg PO tid ×10 days

  - For penicillin-allergic patients: TMP-SMX, 1 tablet PO bid×10 days

  - Amoxicillin/clavulanate (Augmentin) or fluoroquinolones ×10 days for moderate to severe infection

  - If symptoms do not resolve with the first course of therapy, continue for a total of 3–6 wks.

- **Nasal decongestant sprays:** Limit use to 3 days (avoid rebound congestion).

  - Oxymetazoline (Afrin), 2 sprays bid ×3 days.

  - Phenylephrine (Neo-Synephrine), 2–3 sprays bid ×3 days.

- **Oral decongestants:** Pseudoephedrine (Sudafed), 60 mg PO q4–6h.

- **Nonpharmacologic therapy:** Fluids, rest, steam, hot washcloth on face, environmental controls if allergic rhinitis is suspected as a contributing cause, saline nasal spray to decrease edema.

Chronic bacterial sinusitis requires a longer course of antibiotics.

- **Antibiotics:**

  - The same medications as above can be used for 3- to 4-wk courses.

  - Fluoroquinolones can also be used and may have better compliance (once-a-day dosing). However, amoxicillin and TMP-SMX are still considered first-line therapy.

- **Steroids,** either nasal or systemic, can be used to decrease inflammation. This is particularly helpful in patients with nasal polyps.

Fungal sinusitis: Will need hospitalization for IV antibiotics, usually amphotericin B.

- **Surgical intervention:** May be indicated for treatment failures.

When to Refer

- Refer to an otolaryngologist for suspected mechanical obstruction or if the patient has recurrent, difficult-to-control sinusitis that may benefit from surgical intervention.

- Consider referral to an allergist for patients with allergic rhinitis.

- Refer to an ophthalmologist for orbital infections with visual symptoms or ocular signs.

What to Tell the Patient

- Acute sinusitis occurs after viral infections and often clears on its own. If prescribed antibiotics, make sure to complete the entire course.

- Chronic sinusitis requires an extended antibiotic course and may require imaging and/or referral to a specialist for further evaluation and treatment.

SUGGESTED READING

Bisno AL. Acute pharyngitis. *N Engl J Med* 2001;344(3):205–211.

Diagnosis and management of rhinitis: complete guidelines of the Joint Task Force on Practice Parameters for the Diagnosis and Management of Sinusitis. *J Allergy Clin Immunol* 1998;102:6.

Parameters in allergy, asthma and immunology. American Academy of Allergy, Asthma, and Immunology. *Ann Allergy Asthma Immunol* 1998;81(5):478–518.

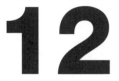

Geriatrics

Clap on . . . clap off . . .

ASSESSMENT OF ELDERLY PATIENTS
Key Issues in Caring for Elderly Patients

As part of a complete history and physical, the following issues warrant consideration in all elderly patients.

Physical health:

- Medical illnesses
- Hearing/vision screening
- Incontinence
- Home safety assessment (e.g., lighting, stairs)
- Balance assessment/fall risk
- Sexual functioning
- Nutrition
- Polypharmacy
- Dental care
- Substance abuse
- Preventive care (e.g., screening, immunizations)

Mental health:

- Cognitive impairment (Mini-Mental Status Exam)
- Depression/anxiety screen (Geriatric Depression Scale)

Functioning:

- Basic activities of daily living (feeding, grooming, ambulation, continence)
- Independent activities of daily living (shopping, cooking, housekeeping, driving, finances)

Social:

- Social support
- Social services needs
- Caregiver burden/placement
- Abuse/neglect
- Finances
- Advance directives/living wills/durable power of attorney

Key Physical Exam

- **Vital signs:** Weight, postural BP.
- **HEENT:** Test vision and hearing, check dentition; remove dentures to look for malignant lesions.
- **Cardiovascular/pulmonary:** Rhythm, murmurs, wheezing, adequate pulses.
- **Abdominal/rectal:** Check for fecal impaction in those with mental status changes or incontinence; in men, check prostate size, especially with urinary retention.
- **Breast:** All women should have clinical breast exams.
- **Muscular/extremities:** Check strength and range of motion; assess standing, bending, turning, walking (especially in those with a history of falls); assess footwear.
- **Neurologic/psychological:** Assess balance and gait; assess for dementia, depression.
- **Skin:** Ulcers (especially in patients with limited ability to ambulate).

EVALUATION AND TREATMENT OF COMMON GERIATRIC CONDITIONS
Immobility

Reduced mobility is *not* normal and is usually secondary to an underlying condition.

- Evaluate for weakness (deconditioning, electrolyte imbalance, anemia), stiffness (Parkinson's disease, osteoarthritis, pseudogout, polymyalgia rheumatica), pain (fracture, cancer, osteoarthritis), and imbalance (previous falls).
- Bed rest can lead to cardiovascular deconditioning, pressure ulcers, muscle wasting, malnutrition, deep venous thrombosis, and pulmonary embolism.
- Provide adequate nutrition. Maintain in the upright position as much as possible each day. Practice range-of-motion exercises (physical therapy), and provide pain control.

Gait Imbalance and Falls

See Table 12-1.

Urinary Incontinence
Causes

- *Acute*: delirium, infection, drugs, psychological issues, polyuria, restricted mobility, stool impaction
- *Chronic*: stress (from pelvic relaxation), detrusor overactivity (urge), detrusor underactivity (overflow), urinary retention (benign prostatic hypertrophy, opioids, anticholinergic medications)

TABLE 12-1.
EVALUATION AND TREATMENT OF RISK
FACTORS FOR FALLS

Risk factor for falls	Suggested evaluation	Suggested initial interventions
Decreased vision	Vision screening	Referral to an ophthalmologist
		Good lighting
Decreased hearing	Audiogram	Cerumen removal
		Hearing aid
Decreased proprioception, balance, sensation	Vitamin B$_{12}$ level, glucose, VDRL	Treatment of the underlying disease
		Good lighting
		Gait training, walking aids
		Appropriate footwear
CNS disorders	Full neurologic and cognitive exam, CT/MRI	Physical therapy, occupational therapy, speech therapy
		Walking aids
Arthritis, muscle weakness	X-ray to confirm arthritis	Strengthening exercises
		Balance and gait training
		Adaptive devices
Bunions, calluses, foot deformities	Careful foot exam	Referral to podiatrist
		Appropriate footwear, orthotics
Postural hypotension	Glucose, BUN, electrolytes	Increased hydration, salt intake
		Lowest effective dosage of necessary medications
		Reconditioning exercises
		Compression stockings
Cardiac, respiratory, metabolic diseases	—	Medications to optimize cardiac and respiratory status
Depression	Depression screening	Cognitive behavioral therapy
		Antidepressant medication
Medications	—	Minimize medications and dosages, or adjust dosing intervals

Evaluation

See Table 12-2.

Treatment

- *Stress incontinence*: behavioral therapy (pelvic muscle [Kegel] exercises, biofeedback), alpha-adrenergic agonists, estrogen, surgical bladder neck suspension.

TABLE 12-2.
EVALUATION OF URINARY INCONTINENCE
IN THE ELDERLY

Symptom/sign	Suggested test(s)
All patients	UA, postvoid residual (>100 mL)
UTI symptoms	UA, urine culture
Urinary retention	Prostate exam (men), BUN/creatinine, renal U/S, cystometry, pressure-flow study (refer to urology)
Polyuria	Blood glucose, calcium levels
Hematuria	Cystoscopy, urine cytology
If no diagnosis is found on initial testing	Urodynamic testing (refer to urology)

- *Urge incontinence*: behavioral therapy (bladder training, pelvic muscle exercises, biofeedback), bladder relaxants, estrogen (if atrophic vaginitis is present), surgical removal of obstruction or other pathologic lesions that may be irritating the bladder.

- *Overflow incontinence*: surgical removal of obstruction, intermittent or indwelling catheterization, treatment for benign prostatic hypertrophy (see Chap. 16, Men's Health).

- *Functional incontinence*: prompted voiding, undergarments and pads, collection devices, bladder relaxants, indwelling catheters, bedside commode.

  - Incontinence may precipitate falls (in an effort to get to bathroom quickly); recommend changing environment (e.g., addition of a bedside commode) to minimize risk.

Pressure Ulcers

- Minimize bed rest (if possible).

- Frequent turns (q2h), air mattress (Kin-Air or Roho mattress), local wound care.

- Meticulous wound care necessary; consider plastic surgery consult for large wounds.

Special Considerations

- The main goals of treatment for a geriatric patient are to identify and correct a reversible illness and to improve functional capacity and overall quality of life.

- Collaborate with the family, physical/occupational therapist, nutritionist, dentist, social worker, home health care worker, and pharmacist. If appropriate, Adult Protective Services and the Department of Motor Vehicles.

- Assess elderly patients in the office and over the phone frequently. If the patient cannot communicate clearly (e.g., hearing loss, aphasia, language barrier), set up an alternate system of communication.

- Discuss advance directives, living wills, durable power of attorney, and code status with the patient and family.

- Referral to a geriatrics clinic for assessment may be helpful.

DEMENTIA
Definition

- Dementia is a syndrome of multiple and progressive cognitive impairments *without a deficit in consciousness.*

- If the patient has an impairment of consciousness, consider a diagnosis of delirium.

- Cognitive functions commonly impaired are learning and memory, attention and concentration, judgment, and social abilities. Personality is also affected.

- Dementia may be progressive or static, reversible or permanent.

Etiology

- Alzheimer's-type (75% of cases) and vascular dementia make up the majority of cases.

Other Causes of Dementia

Symptoms/signs	Suggested diagnosis
Incontinence, gait ataxia, dementia	Normal pressure hydrocephalus
Stepwise progression of dementia	Multiinfarct dementia
Memory loss, confabulation, history of alcohol use or malnutrition	Korsakoff's syndrome
Depressed mood, decreased energy/ motivation	Depression
Fatigue, weight gain, cold intolerance	Hypothyroidism
Ataxia, personality changes, paresthesias, Argyll-Robertson pupil, memory loss	Neurosyphilis
History of HIV	HIV dementia

Key History
Symptoms and Signs

- Difficulty sustaining mental performance, fatigue, and a tendency to fail at novel tasks requiring a shift in problem-solving strategy (initially confined to new things but later spreads to all aspects of daily living).

- Memory impairment (primarily short term), orientation difficulty, language impairment.

- Personality changes: paranoia, hostility, sexually inappropriate (frontal lobe disease).

- Decreased ability to do activities of daily living (e.g., bathing, dressing) and independent activities of daily living (e.g., cooking, shopping, finances).

- Psychosis: Hallucinations, persecutory and paranoid delusions.

- "Sundowner syndrome": Drowsiness, ataxia, confusion, and accidental falls. Occurs in demented patients when external stimuli diminish.

Medications

Review all medications, paying particular attention to opiates, benzodiazepines, anticholinergics.

Family History

Alzheimer's disease, early dementia.

Social History

Living situation, home environment, occupational exposures (e.g., heavy metals), diet, tobacco use, alcohol use, drug use.

Focused Physical Exam

- **General:** vital signs, grooming, wasting
- **HEENT:** hearing, visual acuity, thyroid, carotid bruits
- **Cardiovascular:** rhythm, murmurs
- **Neurologic:** focal neurologic deficits (motor and sensory), unsteady gait
- **Psychological:** mental status exam, evidence of depression

Evaluation

- Rule out reversible causes of dementia in all patients.

- **Labs:** CBC, TSH, VDRL or RPR, LFTs, ESR, serum chemistries (including glucose, Ca, Mg), HIV, UA.

- **Imaging:** Consider CT or MRI of head to rule out cerebrovascular accident, trauma, or tumor (particularly if recent-onset dementia or acute worsening of symptoms).

- Consider lumbar puncture to rule out infection or normal pressure hydrocephalus (be sure to record opening pressure).

- Consider blood and urine screen for alcohol, drugs, and heavy metals (if indicated).

- Chest x-ray.

- ECG.

- Assessment of impairment using a standardized scale, such as the Folstein Mini-Mental Status Exam or the Blessed Dementia Scale (Table 12-3).

TABLE 12-3.
SHORT BLESSED DEMENTIA SCALE

- Begin with the the 6-Item Short Blessed Test (SBT)

This is a shortened version of the Blessed Information Memory Concentration Test. Score 1 point for errors up to the maximum indicated and a zero if correct.

Items	Score	Maximum Error	x	Weight	
1. What *year* is it now?		1	x	4	=
2. What *month* is it now?		1	x	3	=
Memory	Repeat this phrase after me:				
Phrase	John Brown, 42 Market Street, Chicago				
3. About what *time* is it? (within 1 hour)		1	x	3	=
4. *Count* backwards 20 to 1		2	x	2	=
5. Say the months in reverse order.		2	x	2	=
6. Repeat the memory phrase.		5	x	2	=

Total ____

- If time permits then administer the full Blessed Information Memory Concentration Test (BIMC)

INFORMATION   Score

Name ____
Age ____
Time (hour) ____
Time of day ____
Day of week ____
Date ____
Month ____
Season ____
Year ____
Place: name ____
street ____
town ____
Type of place (for example, home, hospital, etc.) ____
Recognition of two persons (one point for each) ____

MEMORY
Personal

Date of birth ____
Place of birth ____
School attended ____
Occupation ____
Name of siblings/name of spouse ____

(*continued*)

TABLE 12-3.
CONTINUED

Name of any town where patient worked/lived   _____
Name of employers   _____
     _____

Non-personal

Date of First World War (1/2 within 3 years)
Date of Second World War (1/2 if within 3 years)   _____
*Monarch   _____
*Prime Minister   _____
     _____

Five-minute recall (score 0-5 points)

Mr John Brown
42 West Street   _____
Chicago

CONCENTRATION (all scored 0-1-2)

Months of year backwards
Counting 1-20   _____
Counting 20-1   _____
     _____

TOTAL: _____

* monarch and prime minister are used as this test was first developed in Britain. They can be substituted by any commonly recognized person (e.g. president)

- Next, gauge several aspects of cognition not included in the Short Blessed:

  - Thought production, form, and content
  - Presence of hallucinations
  - Judgment: "What would you do if you found an envelope with a stamp on it, lying on the sidewalk?"
  - Abstraction: "The grass is always greener on the other side" – what does that mean?
  - Apraxia: Ask the patient to simulate combing their hair or saluting
  - Agnosia: Place a coin in the patient's hand and test recognition

- **Blessed Dementia Scale:** As mentioned before, it is crucial to interview family members as well. This test gauges how the patient's dementia is affecting his or her ability to perform activities of daily living (ADLs).

Circle the number that best rates the changes in memory and performance since the person began having difficulties.

No Loss	Some Loss	Severe Loss	
0	0.5	1	B. Ability to cope with small sums of money.
0	0.5	1	C. Ability to remember a short list of items such as a shopping list.

(continued)

TABLE 12-3.
CONTINUED

0	0.5	1	D. Ability to find way about indoors (home or familiar location).
0	0.5	1	E. Ability to find way around familiar streets.
0	0.5	1	F. Ability to grasp situations or explanations.
0	0.5	1	G. Ability to recall recent events.
0	0.5	1	H. Tendency to dwell in the past.

II. *For each ADL below, choose the <u>one</u> that currently describes the person with dementia.*

EATING

0 Feeds self without assistance.
1 Feeds self with minor assistance.
2 Feeds self with much assistance.
3 Has to be fed.

DRESSING

0 Unaided.
1 Occasionally misplaces buttons, etc. Requires much help.
2 Wrong sequences, forgets items, and requires much assistance.
3 Unable to dress.

TOILET

0 Cleans and cares for self at toilet.
1 Occasional incontinence, or needs to be reminded.
2 Frequent incontinence, or needs much assistance.
3 Little or no control.

III. ***TOTAL SCORE of Blessed Dementia Scale (0-17)*** _____

Reprinted with permission from Blessed G, Tomlinson BE, Roth M. The association between quantitative measures of dementia and of senile change in the cerebral grey matter of elderly subjects. *Br J Psychiatry* 1968;114:797–811.

- Neuropsychiatric testing is often helpful in differentiating dementia from other neuropsychiatric syndromes if it cannot be done clinically.

Management

- Treat any causes of reversible dementia.
- Education of both patients and family members is important for successful management of dementia.
- **Ensure that the patient is living in a safe situation.** If patients need help with independent activities of daily living or activities of daily living, consider:
  - Home health nurse visits for a home safety evaluation (they will assess how appropriate the patient's living situation is for his or her health condition)
  - Meals on Wheels
  - Adult day care programs

- City/county/state division of aging
- Assisted-living facilities
- Nursing home placement
- **Nonpharmacologic treatment** for behavioral problems:
  - Maintain a daily routine and surround patient with familiar people and surroundings.
  - For insomnia, increase daytime activities and decrease daytime naps.
  - For wandering, if possible encourage movement with supervision and conceal doorways.
  - The Alzheimer's Association "Safe Return" program: Patient wears a form of identification with a toll-free number to call in case he or she is found wandering (contact local Alzheimer's Association chapter for details).
- **Medications** can be useful to manage memory loss and behavioral problems.
  - **Anticholinesterases:** May help in delaying cognitive decline and preserving functional capacity for approximately 12 mos in mild to moderately severe Alzheimer's dementia.
    - Tacrine (Cognex), 40 mg PO qid.
    - Donepezil (Aricept), 5 mg PO qd ×5 days, then 10 mg PO qd.
    - Side effects include nausea, vomiting, diarrhea, and insomnia.
  - **Vitamin E,** 2000 IU PO qd, has been found to delay progression to nursing home placement by 4–6 mos.
  - **Thiamine,** 100 mg PO qd, for patients with a heavy drinking history (prevention of Wernicke-Korsakoff syndrome).
  - **Atypical antipsychotics:** These medications effectively control agitation, delusions, and hallucinations.
    - Quetiapine (Seroquel), 25–100 mg PO qhs
    - Risperidone (Risperdal), 1–2 mg PO qd
    - Olanzapine (Zyprexa), 5 mg PO qhs
  - **Typical antipsychotics:** Not used very frequently, owing to strong anticholinergic side effects.
    - Haloperidol (Haldol), 1–2 mg PO bid–tid
  - **Benzodiazepines:** Caution: risk of paradoxic disinhibition in agitated elderly. Not very helpful as monotherapy, but may be helpful as an adjunct for patient's sundowning symptoms.
  - **SSRIs:** Depression and anxiety occur in 40–50% of demented patients.

- Citalopram (Celexa), 10–20 mg PO qd

When to Refer

- Consider referral to a neurologist if consideration revolves around causes of dementia other than Alzheimer's and vascular dementia.

- Consider referral to a psychiatrist if the patient's behavior is difficult to manage.

What to Tell the Patient and Family

- For the most part, dementia is a progressive disease that is not reversible.

- Medications can slow the progression of the disease but are most often used to treat the effects of the disease.

- Encourage the patient and patient's family to discuss the patient's wishes regarding end-of-life care before the patient becomes incapacitated. These issues include

  - durable power of attorney

  - end-of-life care

  - code status

- Refer patients and families to the local Alzheimer's Association (www.alzheimers.org) or other caregiver organizations for information and support.

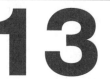 **Gastroenterology**

In one end and out the other . . .

ABDOMINAL PAIN
Differential Diagnosis

Useful to categorize by location of pain (Table 13-1).

Red Flags for Abdominal Pain

- Pain out of proportion to exam → bowel ischemia
- Pulsatile mass → abdominal aortic aneurysm
- Bilious vomiting, high-pitched bowel sounds → bowel obstruction
- Nonreducible hernia → strangulated hernia
- Sexually active woman, positive pregnancy test → ectopic pregnancy
- Peritoneal signs (guarding, rigid abdomen) → peritonitis
- Groin pain radiating to flank → testicular torsion
- Right upper quadrant pain, obstructive LFTs (increased alkaline phosphatase, bilirubin), fever → cholangitis
- Periumbilical to right lower quadrant pain, nausea, vomiting, fever → acute appendicitis

Patients with any red flag symptoms should be evaluated in the ED or admitted immediately!

Evaluation

A thorough history and physical exam are essential to determine necessary workup. *A rectal exam is mandatory for all patients. A pelvic exam is mandatory for all female patients.*

- **Labs:** CBC, Chem 7, LFTs, amylase, lipase, urine beta-hCG (if positive, send serum beta-hCG), lactate (bowel ischemia), UA; consider sending gonorrhea and chlamydia cultures (pelvic inflammatory disease).
- **Radiography:**
  - U/S: for gallstones, ascending cholangitis, ectopic pregnancy, ovarian cyst, hydronephrosis, ascites, abdominal aortic aneurysm.
  - Abdominal obstructive series or upright abdominal film: for obstruction, free air.
  - Chest x-ray: free air under the diaphragm (ruptured viscus), infiltrates, pulmonary edema.

TABLE 13-1.
DIFFERENTIAL DIAGNOSIS FOR ABDOMINAL PAIN

Location	Possible diagnoses
Generalized	Obstruction, peritonitis, SBP, inflammatory bowel disease, diabetic ketoacidosis, sickle cell crisis, porphyria, acute adrenal insufficiency, leaking AAA, ischemic bowel, infection, CHF (bowel edema), lymphoma
Epigastrium	PUD, gastritis, pancreatitis, heart (MI, pericarditis, aortic dissection), pneumonia, pleurisy, subphrenic abscess, GERD
Hypogastrium	Renal colic, ovarian torsion, ruptured ovarian cyst, salpingitis, ectopic pregnancy, endometritis, cystitis, psoas abscess, bowel obstruction, appendicitis, prostatitis
RUQ	Hepatitis, cholangitis, cholecystitis, bowel obstruction, hepatic abscess
RLQ	Appendicitis, ovarian torsion, ovarian cyst, ectopic pregnancy, PID, diverticulitis, renal colic, pyelonephritis, testicular torsion
LUQ	Diverticulitis, colitis, sigmoid volvulus, splenic rupture/abscess/infarct
LLQ	Diverticulitis, colitis, pyelonephritis, ovarian pathology, testicular torsion, ectopic pregnancy, PID, renal colic

AAA, abdominal aortic aneurysm; CHF, congestive heart failure; LLQ, left lower quadrant; LUQ, left upper quadrant; PID, pelvic inflammatory disease; PUD, peptic ulcer disease; RLQ, right lower quadrant; RUQ, right upper quadrant; SBP, spontaneous bacterial peritonitis.

- CT scan: abdominal aortic aneurysm, nephrolithiasis, pancreatitis, bowel ischemia, lymphoma, colitis, diverticulitis.

- Consider esophagogastroduodenoscopy or colonoscopy (peptic ulcer disease, gastritis, carcinoma).

- Consider paracentesis (for spontaneous bacterial peritonitis) in patients with chronic liver disease and/or ascites.

Management

- Consider hospitalization for anyone with red flag signs patients unable to keep fluids down due to vomiting, or patients with difficulty following up.

- Treatment is based on underlying etiology. See chapters for specific management strategies.

- If workup is negative, consider a psychiatric component to the pain (abdominal pain is a common manifestation of somatization).

CONSTIPATION

Definition

<3 bowel movements/wk or prolonged defecation (>10 mins) to complete bowel movement.

Differential Diagnosis

- **Congestive heart failure** (bowel edema)
- **Immobilization**
- **Irritable bowel syndrome (IBS)**
- **Mechanical obstruction** (colon cancer, extraluminal tumor compression, strictures, toxic megacolon)
- **Medications** (narcotics, tricyclics, calcium channel blockers, iron, antihistamines, diuretics)
- **Metabolic disorders** (diabetes, hypothyroidism, elevated Ca^{2+}, decreased K^+, decreased Mg^{2+}, chronic renal failure/uremia)
- **Myopathy** (amyloid, scleroderma)
- **Neuropathy** (spinal cord injury, cerebrovascular disease, MS, Parkinson's disease)

Red Flags for Constipation

- Weight loss
- Use of high-dose laxatives for management
- Anemia, bright red blood per rectum, guaiac positive
- Fecal incontinence
- Abdominal pain
- Family history of colon cancer
- Persistent constipation despite therapy

Unless red flags are present, initially follow conservatively.

Evaluation

- **Labs:** CBC, Chem 7 (increased glucose, increased Ca^{2+}, decreased potassium), TSH
- **Anatomic evaluation** (especially if >50 yrs): colonoscopy, flexible sigmoidoscopy, or air contrast barium enema
- **Abdominal obstructive radiograph:** extent of fecal retention, obstruction, megacolon, volvulus

Management

- **Treat the underlying condition,** if identified.
- **Induce bowel movements:**
  - **Hyperosmolar agents:**
    - Lactulose, 15–30 mL PO qd–bid
    - Sorbitol, 15–30 mL PO qd–bid
    - Polyethylene glycol (MiraLax), 1 tsp (17 g) in water PO qd–bid
  - **Suppositories:**
    - Glycerin suppository, 1 PR prn until bowel movement
    - Bisacodyl (Dulcolax), 10 mg PR prn until bowel movement
    - Senna (Senokot), 1 suppository PR prn until bowel movement
  - **Stimulants:**
    - Bisacodyl (Dulcolax), 10–15 mg PO bid until bowel movement
    - Senna (Senokot), 2–4 tabs or 1- to 2-tsp granules with water or 10- to 15-mL syrup PO qd until bowel movement
  - **Enemas:** tap H_2O enema, 500 mL PR ×1
- Stimulants (either in enema or PO form) intended only for short-term use.
- Soap suds and phosphate enemas are not recommended given potential for mucosal injury.
- **Prescribe a maintenance bowel regimen** for the patient, including
  - **Lifestyle modifications:** daily exercise (walking), development of "daily bowel routine," adequate hydration
  - **Fiber:**
    - Bran (cereals), 1 cup/day
    - Psyllium (Metamucil, Fiberall), 1 tsp in water PO up to tid
    - Methylcellulose (Citrucel), 1 tsp in water PO up to tid
    - Ca^{2+} polycarbophil (Fiber-Con), 2–4 tabs PO qd with water
  - **Stool softeners:** docusate sodium (Colace), 100 mg PO bid
  - **Saline laxatives:** milk of magnesia, 15–30 mL PO qd–bid
- **Avoid magnesium- and phosphate-containing laxatives and enemas in patients with renal failure (can lead to hyperphosphatemia or hypermagnesemia).**

When to Refer

Refer to a gastroenterologist for suspected malignancy or if a colonoscopy is required.

What to Tell the Patient

- A wide variation in bowel movement frequency exists (i.e., patient may not have "constipation").

- Natural gastrocolic reflex promotes bowel movement $1/2$ hr after meals (let nature give the patient a hand).

- Fiber supplementation without adequate fluid intake can make constipation worse.

- Chronic constipation takes a long time to develop and likewise may take time to resolve.

- Stimulant laxatives are not to be used long term (can injure the bowel).

DIARRHEA
Differential Diagnosis

See Table 13-2.

Key History

- **General:** thirst, weight loss (dehydration), fever (infection)

- **GI:** bloating/flatus, cramping (irritable bowel syndrome, cholesterol malabsorption)

  - Duration: protracted acute >14 days (EPEC—enteropathogenic *E. coli, Giardia, Yersinia, C. difficile*)

  - Frequency: persists despite fasting state, nocturnal diarrhea (suggests secretory diarrhea)

  - Volume: >1 L/day (hormone-producing tumors, *Vibrio*)

  - Type:

    - "Rice water" (*Salmonella,* ETEC—enterotoxic *E. coli, Vibrio*)

    - "Bloody" (*Salmonella, Shigella, Campylobacter,* EHEC, *C. difficile, Entamoeba*)

    - "Frothy" (*Giardia*)

    - "Greasy/difficult to flush" (steatorrhea)

- **Genitourinary:** oliguria (dehydration)

- **Social history:**

  - Travel history (travel to Mexico, Third World countries is a risk factor for ETEC, *Vibrio*)

  - Anal intercourse (risk factor for herpes, *Chlamydia,* syphilis, Entamoeba, gonococcus, *Cryptosporidia*)

  - Camping/swimming (*Giardia*)

  - Occupation (day-care setting is a risk factor for *Cryptosporidia, Campylobacter, Shigella*)

TABLE 13-2.
DIFFERENTIAL DIAGNOSIS OF DIARRHEA

Acute (abnormally loose stool of excessive frequency/output [>200 g/24 hrs], present <4 wks)

Viral infection (rotavirus, Norwalk virus, enteric adenoviruses, cytomegalovirus)

Bacterial infection/toxin (*Staphylococcus, Shigella, Salmonella, Campylobacter, Escherichia coli, Yersinia, Clostridium difficile, Bacillus, Vibrio*)

Protozoal infections (*Giardia, Entamoeba, Cryptosporidia, Cyclospora*)

Ischemic colitis

Diverticulitis

Radiation colitis

Inflammatory bowel disease (ulcerative colitis/Crohn's)

Chronic (increased stool production >200 g for >4 wks)

Chronic/relapsing infection (*Clostridium difficile, Giardia*, amebiasis, HIV)

Inflammatory bowel disease (ulcerative colitis, Crohn's disease, collagenous or microscopic colitis)

Steatorrhea

Malabsorption (lactose and sucrose intolerance, celiac sprue)

Diet

Medications (antibiotics, antiepileptic medications, antihistamines, bowel stimulants [metoclopramide] and laxatives, chemotherapy agents, diabetes agents [metformin, acarbose], H_2-antagonists, antacids [Mg-containing], HMG-CoA reductase inhibitors, HIV drugs)

Laxative abuse

Ischemic colitis

Functional (irritable) bowel disease

Endocrine abnormalities (hyperthyroidism, diabetes, pancreatic insufficiency)

Hormone-producing tumors (gastrinoma, VIPoma, carcinoid syndrome)

Postsurgical (gastrectomy, short bowel syndrome)

Colon cancer

- Sick contacts
- Community outbreak (risk factor for food poisoning, *E. coli*)
- HIV risk factors
- Recent hospitalization or antibiotic use (risk factor for *C. difficile*)
- **Diet:**
  - Before onset of acute diarrhea:

- Undercooked meat (EHEC)
- Berries (*Cyclospora*)
- Fried rice (*B. cereus*)
- Cheese (*Listeria*)
- Improperly handled dairy (*Staphylococcus* intoxication)
- Eggs/poultry (*Salmonella*)
- Foods to consider with chronic diarrhea: increased fiber, sugar/dairy intolerance (*lactose*, sorbitol, fructose), caffeine, alcohol

Focused Physical Exam

- **General:** weight loss, fever
- **HEENT:** mucous membranes (moistness), oral lesions (inflammatory bowel disease), scleral icterus, goiter
- **Abdominal:** tenderness, peritoneal signs (*C. difficile*, EHEC, diverticulitis), pain out of proportion to exam (ischemic colitis)
- **Rectal:** lesions, masses, stool color/consistency, stool guaiac
- **Extremities:** edema (malabsorption)
- **Neurologic:** mental status
- **Skin:** rashes (pyoderma gangrenosum can be seen with inflammatory bowel disease; dermatitis herpetiformis can be seen in celiac sprue), lesions, tenting (dehydration)

Red Flags for Acute Diarrhea

- Bloody diarrhea
- Duration >3 days
- Severe volume depletion
- Immunocompromised patient
- High fever >38.5°C
- Recent travel to high-risk area
- Severe abdominal pain
- Confusion/prostration

Evaluation

- Pursue immediately if red flags are present or if diarrhea persists (chronic).
- **Labs:** Chem 12 (elevated Na^+, decreased K^+, increased BUN/creatinine with dehydration), decreased albumin (malabsorption), decreased HCO_3 (acidosis), CBC (leukocytosis), ESR, TSH, gastrin, HIV.

- **Stool studies:** fecal leukocytes, *C. difficile* toxin ELISA, stool pH and weight, stool Sudan stain for fat, stool electrolytes.
- Consider calculating the fecal osmotic gap to distinguish between secretory and osmotic diarrhea:
  - **Fecal osmotic gap = 290 − 2([Na$^+$] + [K$^+$])**
    - <50 mOsm/kg = secretory diarrhea
    - >125 mOsm/kg = osmotic diarrhea
- **Stool for ova/parasites** ×3 (if immunosuppressed or suggestive history).
- **Stool culture** for bacterial pathogens (*Shigella*, *Salmonella*, *Campylobacter*): Notify lab if special cultures are needed (*Yersinia*, *Vibrio*, *E. coli* O157:H7).
- **Rectal swab** for gonococcus, *Chlamydia*, *Neisseria* (suspected STD proctitis).
- **Stool wet mount** for protozoa (sexually active homosexuals, recent travel).
- **Flexible sigmoidoscopy or colonoscopy** (with biopsies for melanosis coli, culture, *C. difficile*, colitis as indicated), **enteroscopy** (with small bowel biopsy for colitis, microscopic/collagenous colitis).
- **Consider abdominal CT** (malignancy, chronic pancreatitis).
- **Consider screening stool sample for laxatives,** particularly if all other tests are negative.

Management

- **Treat the underlying cause,** if detected; consider admission if chronic or severe acute diarrhea.
- **Prevention of dehydration** is very important!
  - Gatorade or oral rehydration solution (1/2 tsp NaCl, 1 tsp baking soda, 8 tsp sugar, 8 oz orange juice; dilute to 1 L with H_2O).
  - Consider admission for IV fluid rehydration if diarrhea is severe.
  - Symptomatic treatment with antidiarrheals is indicated except in cases of invasive infectious diarrhea (risk of inducing toxic megacolon). Hold antidiarrheals if history and symptoms are consistent with a possible infectious cause.
    - **Loperamide** (Imodium), 4 mg PO initially, then 2 mg PO after each loose stool to maximum 16 mg/day.
    - **Diphenoxylate/atropine** (Lomotil), 2 tabs or 10 mL PO qid.
- **Most acute diarrhea is self-limited and does not need antibiotic treatment.** However, antibiotics are indicated for selected infectious diarrhea syndromes:

- Empiric **antimicrobial coverage** for suspected traveler's diarrhea: ciprofloxacin, 500 mg PO bid; levofloxacin (Levaquin), 500 mg PO qd; or trimethoprim-sulfamethoxazole (Bactrim SS), 1 tab PO bid ×7 days.

- *Giardia*: metronidazole (Flagyl), 250 mg PO tid ×7 days

- *C. difficile*: Flagyl, 500 mg PO tid ×10–14 days

- *Salmonella:* antibiotics contraindicated unless severely ill, history of sickle cell disease, elderly, very young

- *Amebiasis:* Flagyl, 750 mg PO tid ×10 days, then paromomycin, 500 mg PO tid ×7 days, or iodoquinol, 650 mg PO tid ×20 days to eliminate trophozoites

- *E. coli* O157:H7: avoid antibiotics (may increase risk or worsen hemolytic-uremic syndrome)

- **Dietary modifications** for patients with osmotic diarrhea:

  - Avoid milk (substitute soy milk or product with lactose already broken down, e.g., LactAid), lactose-containing products, caffeine, alcohol, high-fiber diet, fruit juices.

  - Take an exogenous source of lactase (LactAid) before ingesting dairy products or select products that already contain them.

When to Refer

Refer to a gastroenterologist if

- The diagnosis is not clear.

- Diarrhea persists despite therapy.

- Malignancy, ischemic colitis, or inflammatory bowel disease is suspected.

- There is an indication for colonoscopy and biopsy.

Patients with ischemic colitis require referral to a surgeon.

What to Tell the Patient

- Most acute infectious diarrhea is self-limited and will not need specific therapy.

- Chronic diarrhea is very troublesome; if the underlying cause cannot be corrected, symptomatic therapy with antidiarrheals can be an effective treatment.

- Raising fluid intake to avoid dehydration during episodes of diarrhea is extremely important.

- Finish antibiotic courses as prescribed, because some organisms can be very difficult to eradicate.

DYSPEPSIA

Definition

Persistent or recurrent pain or discomfort located in the upper abdomen.

Etiology

Idiopathic (60%)

Essential, functional, or nonulcer dyspepsia

Organic (40%)

- Peptic ulcer disease (15–25%)
- GERD (5–15%)
- Gastroparesis (diabetic)
- Drugs (e.g., NSAIDs, ASA, antibiotics, alcohol)
- Carbohydrate malabsorption (lactose, sorbitol, mannitol)
- Malignancy (gastric, pancreatic) (<2%)
- Endocrine (parathyroid, diabetes)
- Vascular (intestinal ischemia)
- Connective tissue disease
- Biliary tract disease
- Pregnancy
- Postsurgical
- Psychiatric disorders

Key History/Focused Physical Exam

- **General:** weight loss (malignancy)
- **GI:** nausea, vomiting, melena, hematochezia, early satiety (malignancy), bloating, postprandial fullness, pain relationship to eating, nocturnal pain, tenderness (epigastric, right upper quadrant), masses
- **Psychiatric history:** depression, anxiety (associated with functional bowel disorders)

Red Flags for Dyspepsia

- Age >45
- Dysphagia/odynophagia
- Recent change/worsening symptoms
- Cancer risk factors (smoking, family history, alcohol)
- Failed empiric treatments

- Significant NSAID use
- Early satiety
- Anorexia/weight loss
- Recurrent vomiting
- Iron-deficient anemia (guaiac positive)
- Jaundice/elevated LFTs

Evaluation

- See Fig. 13-1.
- **Initial labs:** chem 12 (LFTs, Ca^{2+}), CBC; consider TSH.
- **Consider *Helicobacter pylori* testing:**
  - *H. pylori* qualitative ELISA serum IgG or urea breath testing.
  - CLO testing can be done if endoscopy is being performed.
  - Role of *H. pylori* in nonulcer dyspepsia is still unclear, with recent trials having conflicting results. However, treatment of *H. pylori* is usually recommended if present; therefore, testing is reasonable.
- **Endoscopy:** Indicated immediately if red flags are present; otherwise, see Fig. 13-1.

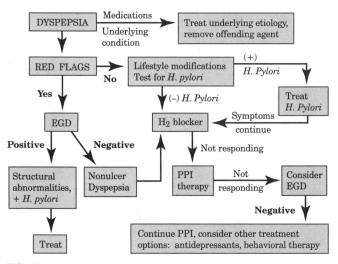

FIG. 13-1.
Algorithm for dyspepsia evaluation. EGD, esophagogastroduodenoscopy; PPI, proton pump inhibitor.

Management

- **Treat underlying condition** if identified; otherwise see Fig. 13-1.

- **Lifestyle modifications:** Avoidance of alcohol, tobacco, and caffeine.

- **Eradicate *H. pylori*** if present, although there is no conclusive evidence that treatment of *H. pylori* improves nonulcer dyspepsia (recent trials are conflicting).

  - Many regimens have been proven effective to eradicate *H. pylori*.

  - One of the most convenient regimens is lansoprazole (Prevacid), 30 mg PO bid, or omeprazole (Prilosec), 20 mg PO bid + clarithromycin (Biaxin), 500 mg PO bid + amoxicillin (Amoxil), 1g PO bid ×14 days (PrevPac). Eradication is achieved in 80–86% of patients.

- **For NSAID-induced dyspepsia:**

  - Stop the medication if possible.

  - If treatment with NSAIDs is necessary, add an acid suppressant (H_2-blocker or proton pump inhibitor [PPI]) or misoprostol (contraindicated in pregnant patients).

  - There is no indication to repeat endoscopy if a first endoscopy was recently negative (unless a new red flag develops).

When to Refer

Refer to gastroenterologist for

- Any red flags
- Endoscopy
- Lack of response to treatment

What to Tell the Patient

- Dyspepsia can be caused by a number of diseases and medications, but in most cases there is no underlying etiology (i.e., most cases of dyspepsia fall into the idiopathic category).

- If *H. pylori* is positive, treatment is necessary to eradicate it; it is associated with gastric ulcer formation. However, eradication of *H. pylori* may not cure the dyspepsia.

- Upper endoscopy may be necessary to rule out structural abnormalities or other causes of dyspepsia.

GASTROESOPHAGEAL REFLUX DISEASE
Key History

- **HEENT:** dental decay/cavities, ear pain, hiccups, chronic hoarseness
- **Cardiovascular:** chest pain or "burning"

- **Pulmonary:** chronic cough, asthma, bronchitis
- **GI:** heartburn, regurgitation (worse when supine/recumbent or bending over), water brash (bitter/salty taste in mouth), nausea and vomiting
- **Genitourinary:** reflux dyspareunia
- **Medical history:** connective tissue diseases (scleroderma), diabetes, hiatal hernia
- **Diet:** foods that relax lower esophageal sphincter (fatty foods, alcohol, chocolate), spicy foods, acidic foods (cola, coffee, tea, citrus, tomato), late-night meals
- **Medications:** calcium channel blockers, anticholinergics, nitrates, sedatives, theophylline, bisphosphonates (alendronate), NSAIDs, KCl; over-the-counter medications
- **Social history:** alcohol abuse, smoking

Focused Physical Exam
- **General:** weight loss
- **HEENT:** dental decay, halitosis
- **Pulmonary:** wheezing
- **GI:** epigastric tenderness, abdominal pain, masses
- **Rectal:** guaiac positive stool

Red Flags for GERD
- Cancer risk factors (smoking, family history, alcohol)
- Advanced age at presentation
- Dysphagia/odynophagia
- Long-standing history of symptoms
- Recent change or worsening of symptoms
- Anorexia, weight loss
- GI bleeding, iron-deficiency anemia
- Recurrent vomiting or hematemesis

Evaluation
See Fig. 13-2.
- **Labs:** CBC (iron-deficiency anemia)
- **Endoscopy** is recommended for
  - Any patient with a red flag (see above)

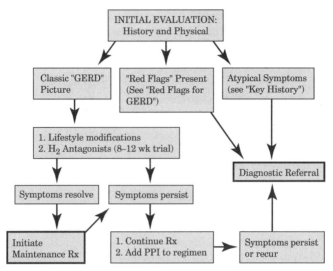

FIG. 13-2.
Algorithm for GERD evaluation. PPI, proton pump inhibitor; Rx, prescription. (Adapted from Treatment of gastroesophageal reflux disease: use of algorithms to aid in management. *Am J Gastro* 1999;94:S3–S10.)

- Patients with atypical GERD symptoms (e.g., cough, asthma, hoarseness, chest pain, aphthous ulcers, hiccups, or dental erosions)
- Patients who are refractory to treatment or need medications for prolonged periods of time
- Any patient with symptoms for >5 yrs for surveillance for Barrett's esophagus

- **24-hr esophageal pH monitoring:**
  - Most sensitive evaluation for reflux
  - Consider in refractory patients with negative endoscopy or atypical symptoms who have failed empiric therapy
  - Identifies temporal associations between activities and reflux
- **Barium swallow:**
  - Limited ability to confirm GERD
  - May provide info on strictures/rings/webs in those with dysphasia as well as GERD
- *Symptoms are not necessarily reflective of disease severity* (Barrett's esophagus, peptic stricture may occur with little to no symptoms; conversely, may have severe symptoms with no pathologic abnormality).

Management

Lifestyle Modifications

- Dietary changes are extremely important.
  - Eat less fat, avoid irritants (e.g., tomato, citrus, coffee, cola, chocolate).
  - No eating 2–3 hrs before bedtime.
  - Eat small meals and avoid lying down after eating.
- Elevate head of bed 6 in. (use concrete block under bed or foam wedge under pillow).
- Stop smoking; avoid alcohol.
- Lose weight.

Medications

Begin an empiric trial of 8–12 wks with medication (H_2-blocker or PPI).

- **H_2 receptor antagonists** (mainstay of GERD therapy for patients with mild to moderate symptoms):
  - Ranitidine (Zantac), 150 mg PO bid.
  - Famotidine (Pepcid), 20–40 mg PO bid.
  - Cimetidine (Tagamet), 400 mg PO bid.
  - Nizatidine (Axid), 150–300 mg PO bid.
  - Take prior to meal or qhs (to block basal acid).
- **PPIs** can be used if H_2-blockers fail as initial therapy, especially in patients with severe symptoms:
  - Lansoprazole (Prevacid), 15–30 mg PO qd–bid.
  - Omeprazole (Prilosec), 20–40 mg PO qd.
  - Esomeprazole (Nexium), 20–40 mg PO qd–bid.
  - Take 30 mins before meals.
  - Initiate if evidence of laryngeal reflux exists.
  - Maintenance therapy is generally with H_2-blockers.
  - For severe GERD, may try PPI qd–bid and H_2-blocker qhs.
- **Antireflux surgery** (fundoplication) is an option for endoscopically proven pathology (erosive esophagitis, strictures, Barrett's esophagus) or symptoms refractory to lifestyle and maximal medical intervention.

When to Refer

- Refer to a gastroenterologist for endoscopy.
- Patients with Barrett's esophagus should be followed by a gastroenterologist for periodic endoscopic surveillance and biopsies.

What to Tell the Patient

- Lifestyle modifications are simple and often effective in controlling heartburn.

- The majority of patients eventually find relief once the treatment regimen is optimized.

- Complications of GERD: ulcers, esophageal strictures, iron-deficiency anemia, and Barrett's esophagus.

- Patients are not alone (>60 million Americans experience GERD on a monthly basis).

IRRITABLE BOWEL SYNDROME
Definition

A disorder characterized by altered bowel habits and abdominal pain in the absence of organic disease.

Key History/Focused Physical Exam

- **General:** weight loss, fever, chills, sweats, anorexia (all absent in IBS)
- **GI:**
  - Abdominal discomfort (cramping; or poorly localized, migratory)
  - Intensity, onset, radiation, duration, frequency of symptoms
  - Association to bowel movements (relief) and meals (worse 1–2 hrs after)
  - Exacerbators (stress, food, hormones)
  - Stool pattern: constipation, diarrhea, mucus, urgency
  - Bloating, dyspepsia, nausea and vomiting, heartburn
- **Genitourinary:** endometriosis, frequency, dyspareunia, sexual dysfunction
- **Medical history:** fibromyalgia, interstitial cystitis, previous sexual/physical abuse, endometriosis
- **Psychiatric:** depression, anxiety
- **Medications:** laxatives, lactulose, constipating medications (see Constipation)
- **Social history:** diet (lactose, fructose, sorbitol)

Red Flags for IBS

Generally **absent** in IBS:

- Onset >50 yrs
- Family history of cancer, inflammatory bowel disease, celiac sprue
- Persistent diarrhea with dehydration

- Anorexia/weight loss
- Severe constipation/fecal impaction
- Pain awakening from sleep/nocturnal diarrhea
- GI bleed (guaiac positive), rectal bleeding
- Steadily worsening symptoms
- Anemia

Evaluation

- See Table 13-3 for diagnostic criteria.
- **Determine predominant symptom:** constipation, diarrhea, or abdominal pain.
- **Labs:**
  - CBC, Chem 12, TSH, ESR.
  - Lab abnormalities unusual in IBS.
- **Stool studies:** For diarrhea-predominant symptoms, consider stool for ova/parasites and enzyme immunoassay for *Giardia*, 24-hr stool collection (usually <300 g/24 hrs in IBS), and stool alkalinization (if stool collection >300 g, evaluate for laxative abuse).

TABLE 13-3.
ROME II DIAGNOSTIC CRITERIA FOR
IRRITABLE BOWEL SYNDROME

A. ≥12 wks (not necessarily consecutive) in the preceding 12 mos of abdominal discomfort or pain that has two of three features:

Relieved with defecation

Onset associated with change in frequency of stool

Onset associated with change in appearance of stool

B. Symptoms that cumulatively support the diagnosis of IBS:

Abnormal stool frequency (>3/day or <3/wk)

Abnormal stool form (lumpy/hard or loose/watery)

Abnormal stool passage (straining, urgency, incomplete evacuation)

Passage of mucus

Bloating or feeling of abdominal distention

Adapted from Thompson NG, Longstretch G, Drossman DA, et al. Functional bowel disorder and functional abdominal pain. In: Drossman DA, Corazziari E, Tally NJ, et al. (eds). *Rome II: The functional gastrointestinal disorders,* 2nd ed. McLean, VA: Degnon Associates, 2000:351–432.

- Consider **anatomic evaluation, especially if red flags are present:** flexible sigmoidoscopy (patient <50 yrs) or colonoscopy (patient >50 yrs) and esophagogastroduodenoscopy.

Management

If the patient does not have any red flags, it is reasonable to treat the patient in a primary care setting. Treatment is based on symptomatology.

- **For abdominal pain:**
  - **Anticholinergics:** hyoscyamine (Levsin), 0.125–0.25 mg PO/SL qid (take qAc and qhs) or dicyclomine (Bentyl), 20–40 mg PO qid.
  - **Tricyclic antidepressants:** amitriptyline (Elavil), nortriptyline (Pamelor), desipramine, 25–75 mg PO qd. (Effective at doses lower than antidepressant dose.)
  - **COX-2 inhibitors:** rofecoxib (Vioxx), 12.5–25 mg PO qd, or celecoxib (Celebrex), 200 mg PO qd.

- **For diarrhea:**
  - **Dietary modifications:** Limit caffeine, alcohol, fatty foods, flatulogenic vegetables (beans, cabbage), sorbitol, and dairy products.
  - **Antidiarrheals:** Loperamide, 2 mg PO bid–qid, or diphenoxylate (2.5 mg)/atropine (0.025 mg) 2 tabs PO qid.
  - See also Diarrhea.

- **For constipation:**
  - **Dietary modifications:** Limit constipating foods and increase fiber in diet.
  - **Fiber supplements:** Psyllium, 1 tsp in water PO qd–tid, etc.
  - **Laxatives and stool softeners:** Docusate, 100 mg PO bid, etc.
  - See also Constipation.

- Assess response to treatment in 4 wks.

- A **psychosocial assessment** may be useful in treating the patient.

When to Refer

Refer to a gastroenterologist if the patient has any red flags or is not responding to treatment.

What to Tell the Patient

- IBS is a real disorder with studies documenting increased sensitivity of the bowel wall in persons who have it.

- In IBS, the bowel can overreact to stress and certain food, manifesting as diarrhea or constipation, bloating, and/or discomfort.

- An emphasis on prevention is essential to maximizing function, and treatment often requires a multidisciplinary approach (nutrition, medicine, psychiatry).

- Total cure is not the treatment goal; like many chronic illnesses, symptom control and improved daily functioning are the goals.

SUGGESTED READING

American Gastroenterological Association Medical Position Statement: Evaluation of Dyspepsia. *Gastroenterology* 1998;114:579–581.

DeVault KR, Castell DO. Practice Parameters Committee of the American College of Gastroenterology: Updated guidelines for the diagnosis and treatment of gastroesophageal reflux disease. *Am J Gastroenterol* 1999;94:1434–1442.

Donowitz M, Kokke F, Saidi R. Evaluation of patients with chronic diarrhea. *N Engl J Med* 1995;332:725–729.

Fass R, Langstreth GF, et al. Evidence- and consensus-based practice guidelines for the diagnosis of irritable bowel syndrome. *Arch Intern Med* 2001;161:2081–2088.

Fisher RS, Parkman HP. Management of nonulcer dyspepsia. *N Engl J Med* 1998;339:1376–1381.

Katz PO. Treatment of gastroesophageal reflux disease: use of algorithms to aid in management. *Am J Gastroenterol* 1999;94(11):S3–S10.

Lassen AT, Peterson FM, et al. *H. pylori* test and eradicate vs. prompt endoscopy for management of dyspeptic patients: a randomized trial. *Lancet* 2000;356:455–460.

Romero Y, Evans JM, et al. Constipation and fecal incontinence in the elderly population. *Mayo Clin Proc* 1996;71:81–92.

Thompson NG, Longstretch G, Drossman DA, et al. Functional bowel disorder and functional abdominal pain. In: Drossman DA, Corazziari E, Tally NJ, et al. (eds.), *Rome II: The functional gastrointestinal disorders,* 2nd ed. McLean, VA: Degnon Associates, 2000; 351–432.

Talley NJ, Silverstein MD, et al. AGA technical review: evaluation of dyspepsia. *Gastroenterology* 1998;114:582–595.

14 Hematology

I'm not afraid of a little blood . . .

ANEMIA

Definition

A clinical condition resulting in decreased red blood cell mass, typically the result of underlying disease process.

Differential Diagnosis

See Table 14-1.

Key History

- **Symptoms:** weakness, fatigue, cold intolerance
- **Pulmonary:** shortness of breath, dyspnea on exertion
- **Cardiovascular:** angina, palpitations
- **GI:** hematochezia, melena, hematemesis, coffee ground emesis (GI bleeding)
- **Genitourinary:** menorrhagia, metrorrhagia (iron deficiency)
- **Neurologic:** increased falls, paresthesias (vitamin B_{12} deficiency)

Medical history:

- Bleeding diathesis
- Hemoglobinopathies (thalassemia/sickle cell disease)
- Chronic infectious/inflammatory conditions (anemia of chronic disease)
- Valve replacement (hemolysis), chronic renal failure (anemia of chronic disease)
- Endocrine disorders (hypothyroidism)
- Cancer
- Atrophic gastritis
- Gastrectomy/terminal ileum resection (vitamin B_{12} deficiency)

Family history:

- Ethnicity (African-American, Mediterranean/Middle-Eastern origin)
- History of sickle cell disease, thalassemia, glucose 6-phosphate dehydrogenase deficiency

TABLE 14-1.
DIFFERENTIAL DIAGNOSIS OF ANEMIA

Microcytic (MCV <80)

Iron deficiency: Blood loss (GI tract, menses), malabsorption (gastrectomy), inadequate intake, deficient absorption, increased requirement (pregnancy)

Lead (Pb) poisoning

Sideroblastic anemia

Thalassemia

Anemia of chronic disease: Cancer, inflammation/infection, liver disease

Normocytic (MCV 80–100)

Reticulocytosis: Hemolysis (immune/nonimmune), hereditary spherocytosis, paroxysmal nocturnal hemoglobinuria

Reticulocytopenia: Aplastic anemia, erythrocyte aplasia, chronic renal failure, endocrine disorders (hypothyroidism), anemia of chronic disease, myelophthisis/myelodysplasia

Macrocytic (MCV >100)

Megaloblastic: Folate deficiency, vitamin B_{12} deficiency, drugs (e.g., methotrexate, phenytoin)

Nonmegaloblastic:

  Reticulocytosis: Hemolysis, blood loss

  Reticulocytopenia: Alcohol abuse, liver disease, hypothyroidism, myelodysplasia

MCV, mean cell volume.

- Hereditary spherocytosis
- Hereditary sideroblastic anemia

Medications:

- Chemotherapeutic agents, chloramphenicol (Chloromycetin), phenytoin (Dilantin), azidothymidine (Retrovir)

Social history:

- Vegan diet (B_{12} deficiency), lack of green vegetables (folate deficiency)
- Inability to cook for oneself (elderly); pica suggests iron deficiency
- Residence in old house (lead poisoning)
- Alcohol use

Focused Physical Exam

- **Skin:** jaundice (hemolysis), koilonychia ("spoon nails"—iron deficiency)

- **HEENT:**
  - Pallor/icterus
  - Atrophic glossitis (red, smooth tongue—vitamin B_{12} deficiency), angular cheilitis, mucous membrane bleeding
- **Cardiovascular:** tachycardia, systolic ejection murmur
- **Abdominal:** hepatomegaly/splenomegaly
- **Lymphatic:** lymphadenopathy (malignancy)
- **Extremities:** cool, cyanosis, diminished peripheral pulses
- **Rectal:** hemoccult stool (GI blood loss, malignancy)
- **Neurologic:** paresthesias ("stocking-glove" distribution), decreased vibratory/position sense, clumsiness, ataxia (vitamin B_{12} deficiency)

Evaluation

- **Initial lab evaluation:**
  - **CBC** [Hb, Hct, platelet count and RBC indices (RDW, MCV/MCH)].
  - **Reticulocyte (retic) count** (important in assessment of normocytic anemia): Must correct for degree of anemia to determine the adequacy of bone marrow response.

    $Retic_{corrected} = (retic\ count) \times (Hct_{observed}/Hct_{normal})$

    <2 = inadequate response with anemia

    2–3 = borderline response with anemia

    >3 = adequate response with anemia
  - **Peripheral smear** (microscopic): See Table 14-2.

For microcytic anemia (decreased MCV):

- Iron studies (ferritin, serum Fe, total iron-binding capacity, % saturation)
- Also consider serum Pb level, Hb electrophoresis (thalassemia, sickle cell disease)

For normocytic anemia (normal MCV):

- **Elevated reticulocyte count:**
  - **Hemolysis evaluation:** lactate dehydrogenase, haptoglobin, indirect bili, urine hemosiderin (all increase with hemolysis), peripheral smear (schistocytes, helmet cells)
  - **Coombs' test:** direct (Ab to RBC surface), indirect (serum anti-RBC Abs)

TABLE 14-2.
LAB FINDINGS IN MICROCYTIC ANEMIA

Test	Iron deficiency	Lead poisoning	Sideroblastic anemia	Chronic disease	Thalassemia
Ferritin	Decreased (<100 µg/L)	Increased	Increased	Increased	Normal/increased
Serum iron	Decreased	Increased	Increased	Decreased	Normal/increased
TIBC	Increased	Normal	Normal	Decreased	Normal/decreased
% Saturation	Decreased	Increased	Increased	Decreased	Normal/increased
Peripheral smear	Microcytes, hypochromic RBCs; anisocytosis	Basophilic stippling	Basophilic stippling; dimorphic population	Microcytes	Basophilic stippling; target cells
Bone marrow	Decreased/absent iron	Normal	Ringed sideroblasts	Normal/increased iron	Normal/increased iron; sideroblasts
Miscellaneous	Increased RDW (early)	Increased serum lead	—	—	Hemoglobin electrophoresis

RDW, RBC distribution width; TIBC, total iron-binding capacity.

- **Osmotic fragility** (hereditary spherocytosis, also spherocytes on peripheral smear)

- **Enzymes:** glucose 6-phosphate dehydrogenase, pyruvate kinase

- **Decreased reticulocyte count:**

  - **Labs:** BUN/creatinine; TSH (hypothyroidism), HIV.

  - A bone marrow biopsy is often needed to rule out aplastic anemia, myelodysplasia, or myelophthisis.

- **For macrocytic anemia (increased MCV):**

  - **Megaloblasts, hypersegmented polymorphonuclear neutrophils.** Check vitamin B_{12} level (decreased), serum folate/RBC folate level (decreased).

    - If diagnosis is uncertain, check homocysteine and methylmalonate levels (homocysteine level elevated in folate and vitamin B_{12} deficiency; methylmalonate level elevated in B_{12} deficiency only).

  - **Decreased retic count:** Check TSH (hypothyroidism), LFTs (alcohol abuse, liver disease).

  - **Increased retic count**: For normocytic anemia, elevated reticulocyte count, see above.

Management

Iron-Deficiency Anemia

- **Ferrous sulfate,** 325 mg PO tid (65 mg elemental iron tid)

  - *Side effects*: Nausea, epigastric pain, cramping, constipation, diarrhea (decreased when iron given with meals, although diminishes absorption).

  - *Monitoring therapy:* Increased retic count after 1 wk, increase in Hb of 2 g/dL at 3 wks, correction of anemia by 8–12 wks.

  - If failure to see an adequate response, consider ongoing blood loss, incorrect or incomplete diagnosis, noncompliance, or malabsorption.

- **Ferrous polysaccharide** (Niferex), 50–200 mg PO qd–tid. Fewer GI side effects vs ferrous sulfate, but more expensive.

- **Iron dextran or sodium ferric gluconate** (parenteral):

  - Used in malabsorption or end-stage renal disease, if iron losses exceed maximum oral doses, or if intolerance to oral iron exists.

  - Side effects rare but potentially severe (including anaphylaxis) with iron dextran; potential for anaphylaxis decreased with sodium ferric gluconate preparation.

- **RBC transfusion** (1 U pRBCs should raise Hb 1 g/dL and Hct 3%):

  - Consider in severe anemia, anemia of acute onset (i.e., hemorrhage), or with comorbid conditions (congestive heart failure, coronary artery disease).

  - Evidence suggests that in patients with cardiac disease, there is benefit to transfusion if Hct <30%.

Anemia of Chronic Disease

- Treat underlying medical condition.

- Consider erythropoietin therapy; dosages vary by indication (see Normocytic Anemia below).

Sideroblastic Anemia (Hereditary)

- Consider a trial of vitamin B_6 (pyroxidine), 100 mg PO qd.

- Monitor retic count and hemoglobin for response.

Normocytic Anemia

- Treat underlying condition (renal failure, chronic illness, hypothyroidism).

- Transfuse as necessary.

- **Erythropoietin:**

  - Renal failure: 50–100 U/kg SC 3×/wk

  - Chemotherapy: 150 U/kg SC 3¥/wk

  - HIV/AIDS: 100 U/kg SC 3¥/wk

Vitamin B_{12} Deficiency

- Vitamin B_{12}, 1000 µg IM ×7 days, then q wk ×1–2 mos (to replenish stores), then vitamin B_{12} 1000 µg IM every mo.

Folate Deficiency

- Folate, 1 mg PO qd.

When to Refer

- For bone marrow biopsy, if necessary

- Pancytopenia

- Sickle cell disease

- When considering use of erythropoietin

- For suspicion of aplastic anemia, hemolytic anemia, myelodysplasia, myelophthisis

- Uncertain diagnosis despite lab workup

SUGGESTED READING

Andrews NC. Disorders of iron metabolism. *N Engl J Med* 1999;341:1986.

Massey A. Microcytic anemia, differential diagnosis and management of iron deficiency anemia. *Med Clin North Am* 1992;76:549–564.

Steinberg MH. Management of sickle cell disease. *N Engl J Med* 1999;341:1021.

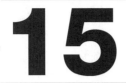

Infectious Diseases

Bring out the bug juice . . .

CELLULITIS
Definition
Usually *Staph* and *Strep* (typically group A beta-hemolytic *strep*). Polymicrobial when associated with lower extremity ulcers in diabetics.

Key History
- **Symptoms:** warmth, erythema, fever, chills, edema
- **History:** trauma, insect bites, lower extremity ulcer, duration of inflammation, progression
- **Medical history:** diabetes, HIV, chronic immunosuppression, peripheral vascular disease

Focused Physical Exam
- **Vital signs:** elevated temperature, decreased BP, elevated heart rate (signs of systemic involvement)
- **Skin:**
  - Extent of area involved
  - Color of skin
  - Margins
  - Bullae
  - Explore wound with sterile probe for wound depth and bone involvement
- **Extremities:** Lower extremity ulcers, lower extremity edema

Red Flags Requiring Immediate Admission
Necrotizing Fasciitis
- Rapidly spreading infection of SC tissue that can lead to septic shock
- Presents with diffuse swelling, anesthesia, rapid progression, bullae, necrosis, elevated creatine kinase on labs
- Requires surgical débridement, IV antibiotics *emergently*

Gas Gangrene

- Often caused by *Clostridia*.
- Presents with diffuse swelling, erythema, bullae.
- Requires IV antibiotics, possibly surgical débridement.

Osteomyelitis

- Can lead to sepsis if untreated.
- Presents with bone pain and fever.
- Suspect if there is exposed bone.
- Requires long-term antibiotic therapy, possible surgical débridement.

Deep Venous Thrombosis

- Has features similar to cellulitis.
- Presents with swollen, warm, erythematous lower extremities; can often palpate cord.
- Requires anticoagulation.

Evaluation

- **History and physical exam** findings to ensure that infection is localized to skin.
- **Blood cultures** if there are any symptoms of bacteremia.
- **X-ray** if you suspect gas gangrene or osteomyelitis.
- **Bone scan or MRI** for suspected osteomyelitis.
- **Lower extremity Dopplers** to rule out deep venous thrombosis (if indicated).
- **Ankle/brachial indices** for suspected vascular insufficiency (if indicated).

Management

Admit patient to hospital for

- Any signs of sepsis, necrotizing fasciitis, osteomyelitis, gas gangrene, or deep venous thrombosis
- Any diabetic with a moderate to severe infection
- Any patient who needs IV antibiotics or surgical débridement

Outpatient Management

- ***Staph* cellulitis:** Dicloxacillin, 500 mg PO qid, or ciprofloxacin, 500 mg PO bid ×3–14 days (depending on severity)

- **Erysipelas (*strep*):** Penicillin V, 500 mg PO qid, or cefuroxime (Ceftin), 500 PO bid ×3–14 days

- **Diabetic foot (mild):** Cefuroxime, 500 PO bid, or amoxicillin/clavulanate (Augmentin), 875/125 mg PO bid, or gatifloxacin (Tequin), 400 mg PO qd ×7–14 days

  - In addition to antibiotics, a strict non–weight-bearing regimen and meticulous wound care are required for proper healing of a diabetic foot ulcer.

When to Refer

- Refer to a vascular surgeon for nonhealing ulcers related to vascular insufficiency.

- Refer to an infectious disease specialist for osteomyelitis.

- Refer diabetics to a foot clinic or podiatrist for orthotics and routine foot care or wound care.

What to Tell the Patient

- Cellulitis is a superficial infection of the skin.

- Finish the entire antibiotic course, even if the redness goes away.

- For diabetics, good foot hygiene is crucial to prevent skin breakdown. Diabetic patients should wear properly fitting protective shoes, check their feet regularly for lesions, and keep their nails trimmed.

- Return immediately if the redness spreads, for fever, or for bone pain.

HEPATITIS
Differential Diagnosis

- **Viral:** Hepatitis A (HAV), hepatitis B (HBV), hepatitis C (HCV), hepatitis D (HDV), hepatitis E (HEV), CMV, Epstein-Barr virus

- **Drugs/toxins:**

  - Acetaminophen (>4 g/day chronically, >7 g/day acutely, especially if combined with alcohol)

  - Antibiotics: fluoroquinolones, synthetic penicillins, ketoconazole/fluconazole, isoniazid

  - Antiepileptics: phenytoin, carbamazepine

  - Cholesterol-lowering agents: statins, niacin, fibrates

  - Substances of abuse: alcohol, cocaine, anabolic steroids

- **Autoimmune hepatitis**

- **Nonalcoholic steatohepatitis (NASH)**
- **Genetic:** Wilson's disease, hemochromatosis, alpha-1 antitrypsin deficiency

Key History
Acute Hepatitis
Presents in three phases

- **Prodromal:**
  - Flu-like symptoms, including fever, malaise, myalgias, arthralgias, upper respiratory symptoms, nausea, vomiting, anorexia (HAV, HCV)
  - Urticaria (HBV)
- **Icteric:** jaundice, right upper quadrant pain
- **Convalescent phase:** resolution of symptoms

Chronic Hepatitis
May be asymptomatic or have complaints related to chronic liver disease (e.g., jaundice, pruritus, ascites/edema, confusion)

Risk Factors
- Travel to endemic areas, especially regions with poor sanitation (HAV, HEV)
- IV drug abuse (HBV, HCV); tatoos (HBV, HCV)
- High-risk sexual behavior (HBV); low risk of sexual transmission in HCV
- Exposure to infected blood products (HBV, HCV), including needle-stick injury or blood transfusion
- Alcohol abuse: may cause alcoholic hepatitis or further liver damage in chronic hepatitis patients

Focused Physical Exam
- **General:** overall appearance, weight gain/loss
- **HEENT:** scleral icterus
- **Neck:** cervical lymphadenopathy (acute hepatitis)
- **Abdominal:**
  - Hepatomegaly and right upper quadrant tenderness (acute hepatitis)
  - Firm/nodular liver and ascites (chronic hepatitis/cirrhosis)

- Splenomegaly (acute and chronic hepatitis)
- **Neurologic:** mental status (encephalopathy)
- **Skin:** jaundice, spider nevi, palmar erythema

Evaluation
Routine Labs

- **CBC:** leukopenia and atypical lymphocytosis (acute hepatitis)
- **Coagulation studies** (PT, PTT, INR): significantly elevated PT = poor prognosis in acute hepatitis
- **LFTs:**
  - Acute hepatitis: marked increase of aminotransferases up to 20× normal
  - Alcoholic liver disease: modest elevation of transaminases, with AST:ALT ratio > 2:1
  - Alcohol abuse: elevated GGT in the setting of AST:ALT ratio of > 2:1

Serologic Diagnosis
Hepatitis A

- Anti-HAV IgM: diagnostic for acute HAV
- Anti-HAV IgG: consistent with previous exposure and immunity to HAV (previous infection or vaccination) in absence of IgM

Hepatitis B

- HBV surface antigen (HBsAg): diagnostic of HBV infection; persistence after acute infection diagnostic for chronic infection
- Anti-HBs: appears after clearance of infection, after vaccination
- Anti-HBc: diagnostic for acute HBV during the window period between clearance of HBsAg and appearance of anti-HBs
- HBeAg and PCR for HBV DNA: markers of viral replication; used to assess treatment response

Hepatitis C

- Enzyme immunoassay (EIA): detects anti-HCV Ab, which is diagnostic of HCV infection.
- Recombinant immunoblot assay (RIBA): also detects anti-HCV antibody; used as confirmatory test for positive EIA in low-risk populations, as false positives may occur.
- Quantitative PCR (viral load) for HCV RNA: used to assess viremia and treatment response; also used for diagnosis in high-risk patients with negative EIA.
- Genotyping is also useful, as it predicts response to therapy.

Hepatitis D

- Anti-HDV antibody diagnostic for HDV; requires presence of HBV infection to contract HDV

Other Diagnostic Tests to Consider in Evaluation

- **Right upper quadrant U/S or CT:** evidence of fatty liver, cirrhosis, or biliary disease.

- **Serum iron studies:** iron overload seen in hemochromatosis.

- **Serum ceruloplasmin:** low levels suggestive of Wilson's disease.

- **Serum protein electrophoresis:** elevation in polyclonal immunoglobulins suggestive of autoimmune hepatitis; decrease in alpha-globulin bands suggests alpha-1 antitrypsin deficiency.

- ANA, anti–smooth muscle Ab: for autoimmune hepatitis.

- **Liver biopsy:** for diagnosis, to assess need for treatment or treatment response.

- Screen for hepatocellular carcinoma in patients with cirrhosis with chronic HBV and HCV with alpha-fetoprotein and imaging (CT or U/S) q6mo–1yr.

Management

Prevention

Hepatitis A

- Vaccination recommended for travelers to endemic areas, patients with chronic liver disease, male homosexuals, drug users, and patients with clotting disorders who receive concentrates.

- Postexposure prophylaxis with immune globulin at a dose of 0.02 mL/kg for all close personal contacts of HAV patients (especially important to treat food handlers, day care workers).

Hepatitis B

- Universal vaccination of infants/children in United States currently recommended.

- Vaccinate high-risk groups: health care workers, IV drug users, male homosexuals, and dialysis patients.

- Postexposure prophylaxis for needlestick injury or newborns of infected mothers, including HBV immune globulin and initiation of vaccine series.

Hepatitis C

- No vaccine currently available; counsel patients about high-risk behaviors.

Hepatitis D

- Vaccinate for HBV.

Treatment

Acute Hepatitis

- Treatment is mainly supportive (rest and maintenance of hydration).

- Avoid hepatotoxic medications and alcohol.

- Patients with evidence of liver failure, such as encephalopathy or prolonged PT, should be hospitalized.

Chronic Hepatitis

- **HBV:**

  - 3–5% of HBV patients will have chronic infection, and 50% of these will progress to cirrhosis.

  - Treatment: Interferon alfa-2b, 5 million U qd or 10 million U 3x/ wk for 4 mos, or lamivudine, 100 mg PO qd in patients with evidence of active viral replication (elevated aminotransferases, HBeAg or HBV DNA in serum).

- **HCV:**

  - 80% of HCV patients will have chronic infection, and 20% of these will progress to cirrhosis.

  - Treatment: Combination therapy with pegylated interferon, 1.5 μg/kg SC qwk, and ribavirin, 1200 mg PO qd for 24–48 wks. Recommended for patients with elevated ALT, detectable HCV RNA, and inflammation on liver biopsy and without contraindications (e.g., severe depression, psychosis, substance abuse, multiple co-morbid conditions). Should be initiated by hepatologist.

- **Liver transplantation** is the only option once end-stage liver disease develops.

When to Refer

Refer all patients to a gastroenterologist with chronic viral hepatitis and elevated ALT levels for possible liver biopsy and treatment counseling.

What to Tell the Patient

- Acute viral hepatitis is often self-limited and will resolve with supportive therapy.

- Avoid alcohol use in the setting of acute or chronic hepatitis.

- Do not start any new medications unless they are first discussed with your doctor, including over-the-counter medications and herbal supplements.

- The treatment available for chronic hepatitis is modestly effective, and there is a high rate of relapse, so prevention efforts are vital. There are support groups available.

- Decrease the risk of spreading HBV and HCV to others: Use condoms during sexual activity and avoid donating blood products or sharing infected drug needles.

CARE OF HIV PATIENTS
Screening

Consider HIV in the following groups:

- Patients with multiple sexual partners
- Homosexual and bisexual men
- IV drug users
- Prostitutes
- Patients who received blood transfusions during 1977–1985
- Patients with known STDs
- Pregnant women
- Patients with active TB
- Hemophiliacs
- Immigrants from endemic areas
- Any patients who consider themselves at risk

Screening tests:

- ELISA, confirmatory Western blot. Consider ordering p24 antigen blood test for patients suspected of having acute HIV infection (8–12 wks after suspected exposure).

- Always counsel your patient about the implications of a positive result, including information about safe sexual practices and STD prevention.

Key History

- **Medical history:** opportunistic infections, other HIV-related complications, previous therapy, depression, other medical problems

- **Social history:** sexual history, drug use, travel history, psychosocial situation

- **Medications:** current medication list

- **Review of symptoms:** fever, night sweats, weight loss, lymphadenopathy, oral lesions, visual changes, swallowing difficulties, diarrhea, rash, shortness of breath, neurologic symptoms, fatigue

Focused Physical Exam

- **Vital signs:** BP, temperature, heart rate, weight
- **HEENT:** funduscopic exam (CMV retinitis), oropharynx (thrush), neck lymphadenopathy
- **Cardiovascular:** murmurs, gallops, rubs
- **Pulmonary:** crackles, wheezing
- **Abdominal:** hepatosplenomegaly, masses
- **Lymph:** axillary, groin lymphadenopathy
- **Genitourinary:** genital ulcers, evidence of STDs, rectal exam
- **Skin:** rashes, Kaposi's sarcoma
- **Neurologic:** complete neurologic exam, including Mini-Mental Status Exam

Evaluation

- **Labs:**
  - **CD4+ count:** Obtain baseline value, then follow q3–4mos.
  - **HIV RNA** (viral load): Obtain baseline value before each change in antiretroviral therapy and q3–4mos thereafter to monitor treatment.
  - **HIV genotyping:** Done to look for mutations that may confer resistance to certain antiretroviral medications. Usually done by HIV specialists.
  - Baseline **CBC, electrolytes, LFTs:** Monitor q3–4mos if on antiretroviral therapy.
  - **VDRL** for syphilis.
  - **Toxoplasma IgG.**
  - **HBV and HCV serologies.**
  - **Fasting lipid panel.**
- **TB skin test:** Reaction >5 mm is considered positive in HIV patients. Patients may become anergic as immune system wanes. Chest x-ray is indicated in this setting.
- **Pap smear** for women ≥1×/yr to screen for cervical carcinoma (may be aggressive in HIV patients).

Management

- For all HIV+ patients, strongly consider **referral to HIV specialist,** as treatment is constantly evolving.
- **Referral to a social worker** for support services and a **dietitian** for dietary guidance.

Antiretroviral Therapy

- Usual antiretroviral therapy includes a combination of nucleoside analog reverse transcriptase inhibitors, protease inhibitors, and nonnucleoside reverse transcriptase inhibitors. *Treatment is individualized.*

- Emphasize to the patient that *absolute compliance* with medications is crucial for successful treatment.

- Side effects: See Table 15-1.

- Drug interactions: See Table 15-2.

Vaccinations

- Recommended for all patients: pneumonia vaccine, influenza vaccine every year, HBV vaccine (if HBV negative), tetanus vaccine q10yrs

- Consider: HAV vaccine

TABLE 15-1.
COMMON SIDE EFFECTS OF ANTIRETROVIRAL THERAPY

Drug class	Side effects
Protease inhibitors	Nausea, vomiting, diarrhea
	Hyperglycemia
	Elevated triglycerides
	Headache, fatigue, depression
	Lipodystrophy
	Nephrolithiasis
Nucleoside analog reverse transcriptase inhibitors (NRTIs)	Neutropenia, thrombocytopenia
	Lactic acidosis
	Peripheral neuropathy
	Pancreatitis
	Elevated liver enzymes
	Depression, insomnia
	Myalgias
Nonnucleoside reverse transcriptase inhibitors (NNRTIs)	Insomnia
	Nausea, diarrhea
	Fever, rash, Stevens-Johnson syndrome
	Elevated lipids
	Elevated liver enzymes

TABLE 15-2.
HIV DRUG INTERACTIONS

Drug class	Interactions
Protease inhibitors (interact with cytochrome P450 system)	Macrolides
	-azole antifungals
	Rifampin
	Beta blockers
	Lovastatin
	Tricyclic antidepressants
	Warfarin
Nucleoside analog reverse transcriptase inhibitors (NRTIs)	Isoniazid
	Metronidazole
	Ribavirin
Nonnucleoside reverse transcriptase inhibitors (NNRTIs)	Amiodarone
	Cimetidine
	Oral contraceptives
	Rifampin
	Warfarin

Opportunistic Infections

- **Viral:** CMV retinitis, HSV, disseminated varicella-zoster virus, oral hairy leukoplakia, progressive multifocal leukoencephalopathy (JC virus [Jamestown virus]), HBV and HCV

- **Bacterial:** bacillary angiomatosis, *Campylobacter* infections, *Salmonella*, pneumonia

- **Mycobacterial:** TB, *Mycobacterium avium* complex, *Mycobacterium kansasii*

- **Fungal:** candidiasis, cryptococcus, histoplasmosis, aspergillus

- **Other:** *Pneumocystis carinii* pneumonia, toxoplasmosis, cryptosporidium, Kaposi's sarcoma, lymphoma

- **Prophylaxis for opportunistic infections:** See Table 15-3.

When to Refer

Refer all seropositive patients to an HIV specialist or HIV clinic.

What to Tell the Patient

- Counsel your patient about treatment options, safer sex practices, and drug and alcohol abuse issues. Many support groups are available.

TABLE 15-3.
PROPHYLAXIS FOR OPPORTUNISTIC INFECTIONS

CD4+ count	Infection	Prophylaxis
<200	PCP	TMP-SMX DS (Bactrim, Septra), 1 tab PO qd or 3×/wk, **or** dapsone, 100 mg PO qd, **or** atovaquone, 1500 mg PO qd, **or** inhaled pentamidine nebulizer, 300 mg q mo
<100	PCP	As above
	Toxoplasmosis	TMP-SMX DS, 1 tab PO qd, **or** dapsone, 50 mg PO qd + pyrimethamine, 50 mg PO q wk + leucovorin, 25 mg PO q wk
<50	PCP	As above
	Toxoplasmosis	As above
	MAC	Azithromycin, 1200 mg PO q wk, **or** clarithromycin (Biaxin), 500 mg PO bid
TB skin test positive **or** prior positive test without treatment	TB	Isoniazid, 300 mg PO qd + pyridoxine, 50 mg PO qd ×9 mos, **or** rifampin, 600 mg PO qd + pyrazinamide, 20 mg/kg PO qd ×2 mos

MAC, *Mycobacterium avium* complex; PCP, *Pneumocystis carinii* pneumonia.

- Remind your patients and their families and friends of the methods of HIV transmission.

- **"Every dose, every day."** Compliance is critical for control of the disease. Patients should be aware that noncompliance can lead to resistant strains of HIV, making the disease harder to treat.

- Especially in advanced disease, discuss how aggressive the patient wants to be with treatment and address code status.

SEXUALLY TRANSMITTED DISEASES
Overview

- Patients with STDs are commonly infected with multiple organisms, so always test and treat for gonorrhea, chlamydia, and syphilis. Strongly encourage HIV testing as well.

- Some STDs are reportable to the local health department.

- Refer all sexual partners to a physician for evaluation and treatment.

TABLE 15-4.
EVALUATION AND MANAGEMENT OF STDS

STD	Clinical features and natural history	Diagnosis	Treatment
Genital herpes (HSV)	**Painful**, grouped vesicles; initial infection may also present with inguinal lymphadenopathy, fever, headache.	Viral culture for HSV	**Acute episode:** Acyclovir, 400 mg tid, valacyclovir, 1000 mg bid, or famciclovir, 250 mg tid ×10 days
	Recurrent episodes likely. Viral shedding (even if patient is asymptomatic).		**Recurrent episode:** Acyclovir, 400 mg tid, valacyclovir, 500 mg bid, or famciclovir, 125 mg bid ×5 days. Must initiate during prodrome or first 2 days of episode.
			Suppression with acyclovir, 400 mg bid if >5 outbreaks/yr.
Syphilis (*Treponema pallidum*)	**Primary:** single, painless ulcer (chancre). Primary disease develops 3–4 wks after contracting disease.	**VDRL** or **RPR** usually positive 4–6 wks after infection. Also used to determine adequacy of treatment, as seronegativity will be achieved in those properly treated after 6–24 mos.	**Penicillin G** benzathine, 2.4 million U ×1 for primary disease or q wk ×3 wks for secondary/tertiary disease (without neurosyphilis).
	Secondary: maculopapular rash involving palms, soles; mucocutaneous disease; condyloma lata; lymphadenopathy.	**FTA-ABS** positive in all stages.	**Doxycycline,** 100 bid ×2–4 wks for penicillin-allergic patients. Consider penicillin densensitization, particularly in pregnant patients.
	If untreated, within 4–10 wks secondary syphilis develops and then enters a latent phase, which can last for years.		

Tertiary: tabes dorsalis, aortic valve disease, neurosyphilis, gummas Tertiary syphilis develops in one-third of untreated patients, usually ≥1 yr after primary infection.	**Darkfield microscopy** of ulcer exudate for treponemes in primary infection. **LP** indicated in patients with neurologic symptoms.	For neurosyphilis, treat with **aqueous penicillin G**, 3–4 million U IV q4 hrs × 10–14 days.
Chancroid (*Haemophilus ducreyi*)	Painful ulcer(s) with bilateral inguinal lymphadenopathy (buboes). Lesions generally appear within 1 wk of infection.	Culture (very difficult organism to grow) or presumptive diagnosis if HSV culture and syphilis testing negative.	**Ceftriaxone**, 250 mg IM ×1; azithromycin, 1 g ×1; or ciprofloxacin, 500 bid ×7 days. **I&D** of large, fluctuant buboes.
Genital warts (HPV)	Soft, painless growths in genital, cervical or perianal areas. May be flat or "cauliflower-like." May have recurrent episodes, even with treatment. Women with genital warts should get yearly Pap smears, as HPV is associated with cervical cancer.	Clinical diagnosis.	Options: **Cryotherapy** **Podophyllin resin:** Apply in office; instruct patient to leave on for 4 hrs and then wash off. **Podofilox 0.5%**, solution bid ×3 days, then 4 days without treatment, then repeat cycle 3–4×. **Imiquimod 5%**, cream 3×/wk at bedtime; wash off 6–10 hrs later until warts resolve. **Trichloroacetic acid** weekly for mucocutaneous lesions.

continued

TABLE 15-4. CONTINUED

STD	Clinical features and natural history	Diagnosis	Treatment
Cervicitis/urethritis (*Neisseria gonorrhea, Chlamydia trachomatis, Ureaplasma uredyticum, Trichomonas vaginalis*)	Purulent vaginal or urethral discharge; dysuria; dyspareunia; postcoital bleeding. In women, can lead to pelvic inflammatory disease and infertility (see below).	**Gram stain:** gram-negative intracelluar diplococci on swab of discharge (gonorrhea) **Wet mount:** for trichomonads. **DNA probe** for GC and chlamydia should always be sent.	**For GC/chlamydia:** Ceftriaxone, 125 mg IM ×1, or ciprofloxacin, 500 mg PO ×1 + doxycycline, 100 mg bid ×7 days, or azithromycin, 1 g PO ×1 for GC and chlamydia. **Always treat for both GC and chlamydia, especially if patient is not likely to follow up.** For *U.urealyticum or Trichomonas:* Metronidazole, 2 g PO ×1 or 500 mg bid ×7 days.
PID	Vaginal discharge, cervical motion tenderness, dyspareunia, pelvic pain, abnormal menses. Often asymptomatic. Usually due to untreated chlamydial or gonorrheal infection. May lead to infertility, ectopic pregnancy.	Clinical diagnosis. Also send cultures for GC and chlamydia.	**Outpatient therapy:** Ceftriaxone, 250 mg IM ×1 + doxycycline, 100 mg PO bid ×14 days, or ofloxacin, 400 mg bid ×14 days + metronidazole, 500 mg bid ×14 days.**Indications for inpatient treatment:** Fever >38°C, WBC count >11,000, peritonitis, abscess, inability to tolerate oral medication.

| Pubic lice (*Pediculosis pubis*) | Pruritus, pubic inflammation. Lice can live on sheets and clothing, so patients can reinfect themselves. | Lice or eggs may be visible on skin and hair shafts. Consider looking at hair under light microscope. | Lindane 1% shampoo (avoid in children and pregnant patients owing to neurotoxicity) or permethrin 1% creme rinse. Advise patients to **launder all bed sheets, clothes, and other linens** in hot (130°F) water, as the eggs can remain on sheets and clothing and lead to reinfection. |

FTA-ABS, fluorescent treponemal antibody absorption; GC, gonococcal infection/gonorrhea; HPV, human papillomavirus; HSV, herpes simplex virus; I&D, incision and drainage; LP, lumbar puncture; RPR, rapid plasma reagent.

Key History

- **Genitourinary:** vaginal/urethral discharge, dyspareunia, painful vs nonpainful ulcers

- **Skin:** rashes

- **Neurologic:** paresthesias, dementia, psychosis

- **Medical/sexual history:** history of STDs, multiple partners, and unprotected intercourse; HIV status

- **Social history:** drugs, alcohol, and prostitution

Evaluation and Management

See Table 15-4.

Difficult Management Situations

- Pregnant patients: Refer to an obstetrician for appropriate monitoring and treatment.

- Patients not likely to follow up: Unless there are contraindications, presumptively treat, especially for gonorrhea and chlamydia.

- HIV testing: Pre- and posttest counseling is required owing to the seriousness of the diagnosis.

What to Tell the Patient

- Most STDs are preventable with use of safe sexual practices. Non-barrier methods do not protect against STDs.

- Untreated STDs may lead to fertility problems for women.

- **All** sexual partners must be identified and told to get evaluated for STDs.

- Consider being tested for HIV and syphilis.

URINARY TRACT INFECTION
Etiology

- *Escherichia coli, Staphyloccus saprophyticus, Proteus mirabilis, Klebsiella pneumonia, Pseudomonas* or *Enterococcus* (in hospitalized patients and patients with catheters).

- **Complicating factors:** male gender, diabetes, immunosuppression, anatomic/functional urinary tract abnormality, nephrolithiasis present, recent hospitalization, catheter, symptoms >7 days.

Differential Diagnosis

- Cystitis

- Pyelonephritis
- Prostatitis
- Vaginitis
- STDs (urethritis)
- Symptomatic bacteriuria
- Urethral irritation due to decreased estrogen (postmenopausal women) or chemicals

Key History

- **General:** fevers, chills
- **GI:** abdominal pain, nausea, vomiting
- **Genitourinary:** dysuria, hematuria, flank pain, foul-smelling urine, vaginal/urethral discharge (STDs, prostatitis)
- **Medical history:** complicating factors (see above), previous antibiotic therapy
- **Neuro:** confusion or acute mental status changes
- **Social history:** relationship to sexual activity

Focused Physical Exam

- **Vital signs:** fever, hypotension, tachycardia
- **Cardiovascular:** tachycardia, murmurs
- **Abdominal:** suprapubic tenderness, rebound, guarding, costovertebral angle tenderness (pyelonephritis)
- **Genitourinary:** for women, pelvic exam, especially if patient complains of vaginal symptoms; for men, rectal exam to examine prostate for benign prostatic hyperplasia, prostatitis

Evaluation

- **Urine dipstick** for leukocyte esterase and nitrites is sufficient for most uncomplicated UTIs.
  - Leukocyte esterase has a 75–90% sensitivity and 95% specificity for detecting pyuria.
  - Nitrites are less sensitive (35–85%) but just as specific (95%). Nitrites can be falsely negative with *Enterococcus*, *Staphylococcus saprophyticus*, and *Acinetobacter* infections.
- Consider **urine culture** if patients have complicating factor or recurrent UTI, or if symptoms persist.
- Consider **further evaluation** for recurrent UTIs:
  - IV pyelogram, voiding cystourethrogram (anatomic abnormalities)

- Renal U/S or CT scan with stone protocol (kidney stones)
- Pelvic exam (vaginal infection)
- Digital rectal exam (benign prostatic hyperplasia, prostatitis)
- Postvoid residual (benign prostatic hyperplasia, neurogenic bladder)

Management

- See Table 15-5.
- Consider hospitalization for IV antibiotics if the patient appears toxic.

TABLE 15-5.
MANAGEMENT OF URINARY TRACT INFECTIONS

Category	Treatment
Acute, uncomplicated UTI	TMP-SMX DS, 1 tab PO bid ×3 days.
	Alternatives:
	Ciprofloxacin, 250 mg PO bid.
	Nitrofurantoin (Macrodantin), 100 mg PO qid.
Recurrent, uncomplicated UTI (>3/yr)	**Treatment same as above.** Consider prophylactic therapy, especially if UTIs correspond with sexual intercourse.
	Prophylaxis: TMP-SMX SS, 1 tab PO qd, or nitrofurantoin, 100 mg PO qd.
	Postcoital prophylaxis: TMP-SMX DS, 1/2 tab or TMP-SMX SS, 1 tab after intercourse.
Acute, uncomplicated pyelone-phritis, outpatient therapy	TMP/SMX ×10–14 days. Send urine culture before beginning therapy.
	Alternatives:
	Fluoroquinolone ×10–14 days if gram-negative organism
	or
	Amoxicillin (Amoxil) for gram-positive or *Enterococcus* species.
	(consider hospital admission for IV antibiotics if patient cannot take orally, looks toxic, or is pregnant or immuno-compromised)

continued

**TABLE 15-5.
CONTINUED**

Category	Treatment
Complicated UTI (male, diabetes, immunosuppression, anatomic/ functional urinary tract abnormality, nephrolithiasis present, recent hospitalization, catheter, symptoms >7 days)	Fluoroquinolone ×7–14 days. Send urine culture before beginning treatment. **Adjuvant therapy/prevention:** Consider intermittent straight catheterization in patients with neurogenic bladder to decrease postvoiding residual and risk of infection. Follow-up culture indicated 1–2 wks after finishing therapy. Consider hospitalization for IV antibiotics if the patient looks toxic.
Catheter-associated UTI	Fluoroquinolone ×10–14 days. Send urine culture before beginning treatment. Not necessary to treat asymptomatic patients with bacteriuria except if pregnant, before invasive procedures, or in organ transplant recipients.
Asymptomatic bacteriuria	None. Treatment not indicated except in pregnancy (40% of pregnant patients go on to develop pyelonephritis), before invasive procedures, or in organ transplant recipients.

When to Refer

Consider referral to urologist for suspected anatomic or functional abnormalities.

What to Tell the Patient

- Remind your patients to complete their full course of antibiotic treatment, even if symptoms resolve.

- Drink at least 6–8 glasses/day of fluids to help keep urinary system "flushed."

- Cranberry juice may be helpful in preventing UTIs.

- For UTIs associated with sexual intercourse, diaphragms and spermicides may contribute to infection, so couples may want to consider alternate birth control methods.

- Call or return if you have persistent fever or UTI symptoms, or if you are unable to take an oral antibiotic because of nausea or vomiting.

SUGGESTED READING

Caputo GM, Cavanagh PR, et al. Assessment and management of foot disease in patients with diabetes. *N Engl J Med* 1994;331(13):854–860.

Lauer G, Walker B. Hepatitis C virus infection. *N Engl J Med* 2001;345: 41–52.

Lee W. Hepatitis B virus infection. *N Engl J Med* 1997;337:1733–1745.

Mundy LM. Skin, soft-tissue, and bone infections. In: Ahya S, Flood K, Paranjothi S, eds. *The Washington manual of medical therapeutics*, 30th ed. Philadelphia: Lippincott Wilkins & Williams 2001;308–310.

Myers RA. Outpatient management of HIV-infected adults. *Postgrad Med* 1998;103(5):219–228.

Pratt D, Kaplan M. Evaluation of abnormal liver-enzyme results in asymptomatic patients. *N Engl J Med* 2000;342:1266–1271.

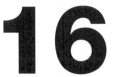

Men's Health

Boys will be boys . . .

BENIGN PROSTATIC HYPERPLASIA
Key History

- For assessment of symptoms, see Table 16-1.

- **Medical history:** frequent UTIs, kidney/bladder stones, instrumentation of the urethra/bladder, bladder/prostate cancer, diabetes, cerebrovascular accident/neurologic disease, colon cancer, metastatic cancer, renal failure, hydronephrosis.

- **Medications:** anticholinergics (tricyclics), sympathomimetics (alpha-agonists, decongestants), antihistamines, diuretics, opioids.

Focused Physical Exam

- **Abdominal:** palpable bladder, suprapubic tenderness

- **Rectal:** estimated size of the prostate, shape, asymmetry, nodules, tenderness

- **Neurologic:** rectal tone, saddle anesthesia (S2–S4)

Evaluation

- **UA** to rule out UTI, hematuria.

- **BUN and creatinine** to evaluate renal function.

- Consider obtaining a **prostate-screening antigen (PSA):**

  - Aids in the evaluation of the size of the prostate.

  - Serves as a predictor of urinary retention and the need for surgery.

  - Establishes baseline to evaluate the effect of treatment (finasteride can decrease PSA), prostate cancer screening (controversial).

  - Decision must be individualized, and potential risks and benefits should be discussed with the patient.

- Consider **postvoid residual** (PVR) to rule out obstruction.

- Consider **renal U/S** if elevated PVR or creatinine.

Management
Lifestyle Modifications
Minimize evening fluid intake; avoid medications that affect urinary function.

TABLE 16-1.
AMERICAN UROLOGY ASSOCIATION (AUA) SYMPTOM INDEX FOR BENIGN PROSTATIC HYPERPLASIA

	Not at all	<1 time in 5	<$\frac{1}{2}$ the time	About $\frac{1}{2}$ the time	>$\frac{1}{2}$ the time	Almost always
1. Over the past month or so, how often have you had a sensation of not emptying your bladder completely after you finished urinating?	0	1	2	3	4	5
2. Over the past month or so, how often have you had to urinate again <2 hrs after you finished urinating?	0	1	2	3	4	5
3. Over the past month or so, how often have you found you stopped and started again several times when you urinated?	0	1	2	3	4	5
4. Over the past month or so, how often have you found it difficult to postpone urination?	0	1	2	3	4	5
5. Over the past month or so, how often have you had a weak urinary stream?	0	1	2	3	4	5
6. Over the past month or so, how often have you had to push or strain to begin urination?	0	1	2	3	4	5
7. Over the last month, how many times did you most typically get up to urinate from the time you went to bed at night until the time you got up in the morning?	Number of times: 0	1	2	3	4	≥5

AUA symptom score = sum of questions 1–7 = _____

From *Benign prostatic hyperplasia: diagnosis and treatment. Clinical practice guide.* AHCPR pub no. 94-0582. Washington: U.S. Department of Health and Human Services, 1994, with permission.

Treatment

Based on American Urology Association symptom score:

- **Mild (0–7):** Watchful waiting; many patients will improve or stay stable without any form of treatment.

- **Moderate (8–19):** Options include watchful waiting for those patients who are not bothered by their symptoms, medical therapy (see below), and surgery.

- **Severe (20–35):** Can start with medical therapy, but patients will likely need surgery.

- **Complications** that require referral for surgery: acute obstruction, urinary retention, chronic renal insufficiency, recurrent UTI, hematuria, bladder stones, hydronephrosis.

Medical Therapy

- **Alpha-1 antagonists:**

  - **Terazosin (Hytrin),** 1 mg PO qhs, titrate over 2–4 wks to maximum 20 mg PO qd; or **doxazosin (Cardura),** 1 mg PO qhs, titrate to maximum 8 mg PO qd. Side effects: orthostatic hypotension (first dose), dizziness, nasal congestion, impotence, somnolence, asthenia.

  - **Tamsulosin (Flomax),** 0.4 mg PO qd, maximum 0.8 mg PO qd (no titration necessary). More selective for prostate. Side effects: headache, dizziness, does not significantly affect BP.

- **Androgen deprivation:**

  - **Finasteride (Proscar),** 5 mg PO qd or dutasteride (Avodart), 0.5 mg PO qd (5-alpha reductase inhibitor). Indicated in patients with large prostates (>40 g). Maximum effect takes up to 6–12 mos to occur. Side effects: decreased PSA (must multiply by 2 for cancer screening), erectile dysfunction.

  - **Bicalutamide (Casodex),** 50–100 mg PO qd (antiandrogen), or flutamide (Eulexin), 125–250 mg PO tid (antiandrogen). Side effects: gynecomastia, breast tenderness, GI symptoms, decreased PSA. Very expensive.

  - **Leuprolide (Lupron),** 7.5 mg IM every mo, or **goserelin (Zoladex),** 3.6 mg SC every mo (luteinizing hormone–releasing hormone agonists). Decreases prostate volume (more than other drugs but may take up to 9 mos for maximal effect). Used primarily in the elderly who are a high surgical risk. Very expensive. Side effects: impotence, loss of libido, hot flashes, gynecomastia, lethargy, decreased PSA.

Surgical Therapy

Indicated for patients with severe symptoms (e.g., transurethral prostatectomy, laser, seeds).

When to Refer

Referral to a urologist is indicated for

- Severe BPH symptoms (for urodynamic studies) or symptoms refractory to medical therapy

- Recurrent bladder stones, recurrent UTIs, recurrent/persistent hematuria, renal insufficiency, elevated postvoiding residual/hydronephrosis

- Elevated PSA on antiandrogen therapy

- Surgical intervention

What to Tell the Patient

- BPH is a common condition due to the benign enlargement of the prostate. It has no relationship to the development of prostate cancer.

- Mild symptoms often improve or remain stable over time.

- Irritative or obstructive symptoms may not always relate to prostate size or respond to therapy.

- For severe symptoms, surgery may be necessary.

ERECTILE DYSFUNCTION

Etiology

Psychogenic

- Sudden onset, young, has spontaneous nocturnal/morning erections

- Performance anxiety, relationship problems, psychological stress, depression

Organic

- Slow progression; no nocturnal erections

- Neurologic (stroke, spinal cord injury, pelvic injury/surgery, diabetic neuropathy)

- Hormonal (hypogonadism, hyperprolactinemia)

- Vascular (atherosclerosis, HTN, trauma, coronary artery disease, Peyronie's disease)

- Drug-induced (antihypertensives, antidepressants, antiandrogens, alcohol, tobacco)

- Systemic disease (chronic renal failure, Cushing's, thyroid disease, diabetes, chronic liver disease, acromegaly)

Key History

Symptoms

- Distinguish between premature ejaculation vs diminished libido vs failure to attain erection vs failure to maintain erection (detumescence)

- Nocturnal erections/spontaneous morning erections

- Erections with masturbation or other partners

- Painful erections

- Breast tenderness, enlargement (hyperprolactinemia, liver disease)

- Intermittent claudication (suggestive of vascular disease)

- Depression symptoms, recent lifestyle events/changes (psychogenic erectile dysfunction [ED])

Medical History

- See Etiology.

Medications

- Anti-HTN (alpha-1 blockers, clonidine, methyldopa, beta blockers, spironolactone, thiazide diuretics), antidepressants (SSRIs, tricyclic antidepressants), anticholinergics, antipsychotics, ketoconazole, cimetidine, nitrates

Social History

- Tobacco, alcohol, drugs, stress assessment, recent events, relationship with the patient's partner, patient's and partner's expectations

Focused Physical Exam

- **General:** elevated BP

- **HEENT:** goiter

- **Breast:** gynecomastia, breast tenderness

- **Cardiovascular:** rate, rhythm, murmurs

- **Abdominal:** ascites, spider angiomata

- **Genitourinary:** decreased pubic hair, penis size, Peyronie's disease (abnormal curvature and shortening of penis during erection), size/consistency of the testes

- **Extremities:** femoral, pedal pulses, bruits

- **Neurologic:** lower extremity motor strength/reflexes, rectal tone, bulbocavernosus/cremasteric reflexes

Evaluation

- **Labs:** UA, CBC, and electrolytes, including glucose, BUN, creatinine, cholesterol, triglycerides, and TSH.

- Check **testosterone level** if hypogonadism suspected; if decreased, check free testosterone, prolactin, and LH.

- Consider **nocturnal tumescence study** (consider referral to a urologist).

- **ECG** if the patient desires pharmacologic therapy.

Management

Nonpharmacologic Therapy

- Remove or decrease dosages of offending medications.

- Decrease alcohol use; cease smoking.

- Consider marital or sex counseling for couples.

Pharmacologic Therapy
Sildenafil (Viagra)

- 25–50 mg PO 1 hr before intercourse (use lower doses with increased age and coronary artery disease). Maximum, 1 pill/day.

- Side effects: hypotension, headache, flushing, nasal congestion, visual changes (color changes, sensitivity to light).

- **Patients must avoid all short/long-acting nitrates (for ≥24 hrs)—can be fatal!**

Yohimbine (Yocon)

- 5.4 mg PO tid; must be taken daily.

- May take up to 2–3 wks for effect.

- Side effects: palpitations, fine tremor, HTN, anxiety.

Alprostadil (Muse) Intraurethral Injection

- 125–250 µg up to 1000 µg; inject intraurethral to 1 in. after voiding.

- Side effects: pain, urethral burning.

Intracavernous Injection

- Alprostadil (Caverject), 2.5–10 µg.

- Titration and teaching must be done in the office.

- Side effects: pain, hematoma, priapism, fibrosis.

- Contraindications: priapism, sickle cell disease, penile fibrosis, penile deformity, penile implant.

Androgens for Hypogonadism

Testosterone cypionate/enanthate, 200 mg IM q2–3wks, or testosterone TTS, 1 patch qd.

External Vacuum Devices

Consider for patients who cannot or do not wish to take medications or injections.

Surgical Options

Vascular surgery and penile implants.

When to Refer

- Refer to urologist for unclear diagnosis, neurologic disorders, Peyronie's disease, and posttraumatic ED.

- Refer to endocrinologist for hypogonadism or other endocrine disorder.

What to Tell the Patient

- ED is a common condition that occurs in men at any age.

- There are both psychological and organic causes of ED.

- For men with psychogenic ED, counseling (both individual and couples) may be helpful.

- Viagra is not for everyone; despite availability over the Internet and other sources, patients must be seen by a physician before being prescribed Viagra. **It can be fatal if mixed with nitrates.**

SUGGESTED READING

Lue TF. Erectile dysfunction. *N Engl J Med* 2000;342(24):1802–1813.
Zippe C. Benign prostatic hyperplasia: an approach for the internist. *Cleve Clin J Med* 1996;63:226–236.

Neurology

Use it or lose it . . .

HEADACHE
Differential Diagnosis
Primary Headaches

- **Cluster headache:** Severe, unilateral orbital or supraorbital pain, ipsilateral conjunctival injection, lacrimation, nasal congestion. Lasts minutes, tends to strike at same time every day, may wake patient from sleep and cause restlessness.

- **Tension headache:** Pressing or tightening quality, bilateral, no aggravation by physical activity, no nausea/vomiting, may have photophobia or phonophobia. Lasts minutes to days. Tends to develop in late morning/afternoon and go away with sleep.

- **Migraine headache:** Unilateral, pulsating pain aggravated by physical activity, with nausea, vomiting, photophobia, phonophobia, aura (e.g., scintillations, scotomata, blurred vision, unilateral paresthesias/weakness).

  - Associated medical conditions: mitral valve prolapse, Raynaud's phenomenon, irritable bowel syndrome, and antiphospholipid antibody syndrome. Triggers include menstrual cycle, pregnancy, stress, sleep deprivation, oral contraceptives, foods.

Secondary Causes of Headache

- **Temporal arteritis:** Pain along temporal artery, dimming of vision in one eye, jaw claudication, age >50, elevated ESR, associated with polymyalgia rheumatica.

- **Subarachnoid hemorrhage:** Sudden onset of headache, patients complain of the "worst headache ever."

- **Subdural hematoma:** Headaches of increasing severity, history of fall or head trauma, increased risk in elderly, history of anticoagulation.

- **Infection:** History of systemic symptoms, neck stiffness, toxoplasmosis, or CNS lymphoma (HIV patient).

- **Pseudotumor cerebri:** Obese young women, papilledema, elevated ICP without other explanation.

- **Mass lesions:** Consider if history of cancer, HIV, or new-onset headaches increasing in frequency and severity.

- **Post–lumbar puncture headache:** Due to low CSF pressure from persistent leakage. Worsens with sitting/standing, improved with lying flat.

Key History

Symptoms	Diagnosis suggested
Bilateral pain, tightening or pressing quality, goes away with sleep	Tension headache
Unilateral pain, nausea, vomiting, photophobia, phonophobia, ± aura, ± neurologic signs	Migraine headache
Associated with menstrual cycle or oral contraceptives	Migraine headache
Nasal congestion, tearing, occurs at same time every day	Cluster headache
Jaw claudication, scalp pain	Temporal arteritis
Stiff neck, fever	Meningitis
Sudden onset of "worst headache ever"	Subarachnoid hemorrhage
Unexplained nausea/vomiting, headaches increasing in severity and frequency	Increased ICP—intracranial mass

- **Medical history:** headaches, malignancy, HIV
- **Family history:** headaches (especially migraines)
- **Medications:** caffeine-containing products, oral contraceptives, nitrates, analgesic use
- **Social history:** exposure to mosquitos, caffeine consumption

Red Flags for Headache

- **Headache onset >50 yrs of age** (temporal arteritis, tumor)
- **Sudden onset of headache** (subarachnoid hemorrhage, arteriovenous malformation, tumor, cerebrovascular accident)
- **Headaches increasing in frequency and severity** (tumor, subdural hematoma, medication overuse)
- **New-onset headache in patient with (or at risk for) HIV or cancer** (meningitis, abscess, metastasis)
- **Headache with fever, stiff neck, rash** (meningitis, encephalitis, collagen vascular disease)
- **Focal neurologic signs** (mass lesion, arteriovenous malformation, stroke, collagen vascular disease)

- **Papilledema** (mass lesion, pseudotumor cerebri, meningitis)
- **Headache after head trauma** (intracranial hemorrhage, subdural hematoma, epidural hematoma)

Focused Physical Exam

- **Vital signs:** temperature, BP, heart rate
- **HEENT:** funduscopic exam (papilledema), tenderness of temporal artery, palpation of sinuses, decreased visual acuity, conjunctival injection, neck rigidity, muscle spasm
- **Skin:** rash (meningococcemia, collagen vascular disease)
- **Neurologic:** mental status exam; cranial nerves; pupils; deep tendon reflexes; sensation; strength; cerebellar signs; Babinski's, Kernig's, and Brudzinski's signs (for meningitis)

Evaluation

- Diagnosis can generally be made from history and physical exam.
- If no red flags are present, a trial of medication is appropriate.
- If red flags are present, or if symptomatic treatment fails, consider
  - **CT scan** of head if suspect mass lesions, hematomas, subarachnoid hemorrhage, cerebrovascular accident, toxoplasmosis, collagen vascular diseases.
  - **MRI** of brain if suspect posterior fossa or brain stem tumors, cerebrovascular accident, or collagen vascular diseases.
  - **Magnetic resonance angiography or cerebral angiogram** if arteriovenous malformations are suspected.
  - **Lumbar puncture** if meningitis or subarachnoid hemorrhage (if CT negative) are suspected.
  - **ESR elevated and temporal artery biopsy** if temporal arteritis is suspected.

Management

Nonpharmacologic Techniques

- Relaxation techniques, adequate sleep, avoiding triggers, decreasing stress levels.

Analgesic Therapy

- Effective for most headaches that cause mild to moderate disability.

- Suggested regimens: ibuprofen, 400–800 mg PO q8h; ASA, 325–650 mg PO q4h; acetaminophen, 1000 mg PO q6h; naproxen, 500–1000 mg PO.

- An antiemetic (e.g., prochlorperazine [Compazine], 5–10 mg PO/PR) can also be added to augment efficacy of the analgesic medication.

Migraine Headache

- **Symptomatic therapy:** As above.

- **Abortive therapy:** See Table 17-1.

- **Prevention:** Consider preventive therapy in patients who have >1 headache/wk or have moderate to severe disability due to their headaches. Commonly used regimens are listed in Table 17-2.

Tension Headache

- Symptomatic therapy with analgesics. Abortive therapies are generally not effective for tension headaches.

TABLE 17-1.
ABORTIVE THERAPIES FOR HEADACHE

Medication	Comments
First-line therapy	Take medication at onset of headache; may be repeated in 2 hrs. Relieves headache in 80% of patients in 2–4 hrs.
Sumatriptan, 25–100 mg PO or 1–6 mg SC, or nasal spray, 5–20 mg	Sumatriptan injections SC may be more effective than oral preparations in patients with significant nausea.
Rizatriptan (Maxalt, Maxalt-MLT), 5–10 mg PO	Contraindicated in patients with uncontrolled HTN, coronary artery disease, history of peripheral arterial disease due to vasoconstrictor effects.
Zolmitriptan (Zomig), 2.5–5 mg PO	Side effects: chest pain, dizziness, flushing, palpitations, MI, hypertensive crisis, cerebrovascular accident.
Other abortive therapies	
Fioricet, 1–2 tabs PO q4h prn	Maximum, 6 tabs/day Side effects: dizziness, sedation, nausea, vomiting
Cafergot, 100–200 mg PO at onset	Maximum, 5 tablets/attack, 10 tablets/wk Side effects: palpitations, anxiety, nausea, vomiting, MI, contraindicated in pregnancy.
Midrin, 2 caps PO at onset	May be repeated qhr as needed Side effects: dizziness, rash, HTN

TABLE 17-2.
PREVENTIVE REGIMENS AGAINST MIGRAINE HEADACHE

Medication	Dosage	Side effects
Propranolol (Inderal)	Start at 40 mg PO bid; may be titrated.	Fatigue, bradycardia, bronchospasm
Amitriptyline (Elavil)	Start at 25 mg PO qhs; may be titrated.	Drowsiness
Valproic acid (Depakene)	400 mg PO bid; may be titrated.	Drowsiness, weight gain, liver abnormalities (must monitor), bone marrow suppression, caution in pregnancy

• Relaxation techniques and stress management can also be effective.

Cluster Headache

• **Oxygen therapy:** 7 L by NC for 10 mins is effective in up to 70% of patients.

• **Abortive therapy** as for migraines (Table 17-1), particularly ergotamine and triptans.

• **Prophylaxis:** Prednisone, 60 mg PO qd ×2 wks, then taper, or verapamil, 80 mg PO bid, or lithium carbonate, 300 mg PO bid.

Temporal Arteritis

• Start **prednisone, 100 mg PO qd, immediately** to prevent vision loss.

• Arrange for a confirmatory temporal artery biopsy.

• Once symptoms resolve and ESR has normalized, can taper steroid dose to maintenance, 10–20 mg PO qd from 6 mos to 2 yrs.

Postconcussive Headache

• Symptomatic therapy with analgesics.

• May take weeks to months to resolve.

Pseudotumor Cerebri

• **Serial lumbar punctures** every few days to few weeks, depending on symptoms, is main treatment.

• Add **acetazolamide,** 250–500 mg PO tid, or **prednisone,** 40–60 mg PO qd, for additional symptom control.

When to Refer

Refer to a neurologist for

- Difficulty with diagnosis
- Headache with focal neurologic signs
- Headaches that are worsening or are not responding to management

Refer to a neurosurgeon for mass lesions.

Difficult Management Situation: Analgesic "Rebound" Headache

- Stems from overuse of analgesics, which precipitate worsening and/ or daily symptoms.
- Advise the patient to minimize use of analgesics (you can help this by prescribing prophylactic medication if necessary).
- To break a headache, patient must stop **all** analgesic medications for 3–4 days, then consider admitting patient to hospital for IV dihydroergotamine therapy.

What to Tell the Patient

- Most chronic headaches are benign, and treatment is symptomatic.
- Overuse of analgesics can exacerbate their headache problem.
- Explain side effects of medications, particularly triptans.
- Avoidance of triggers is the best way to prevent headaches.

TRANSIENT ISCHEMIC ATTACK
Definition

A TIA is defined by focal neurologic symptoms usually lasting <60 mins but always lasting <24 hrs with complete recovery of neurologic function.

- *If patients have signs or symptoms of a stroke, they should immediately go to the ED. (There is a 3-hr window for thrombolytic therapy.)*

Differential Diagnosis

- Stroke
- Cardiac arrhythmia
- Hypoglycemia
- Syncope
- Complicated migraine headache
- Seizure

Key History

- **Neurologic:**
  - Age, timing of symptoms
  - Contralateral weakness or numbness, speech or language dysfunction, visual disturbances (suggests carotid or embolic source)
  - Symptoms of dizziness, vertigo, ipsilateral numbness or weakness, dysarthria (suggests posterior circulation source)

- **Medical history:** atrial fibrillation, rheumatic heart disease, endocarditis, artificial valves, prior stroke/TIAs, hyperlipidemia, diabetes, asymptomatic carotid stenosis, coronary artery disease, hypercoagulable states

- **Social history:** IV drugs (especially heroin, cocaine), tobacco, heavy alcohol use (>5 drinks/day)

- **Medications:** oral contraceptives, over-the-counter medications containing ephedrine or phenylpropanolamine (withdrawn from U.S. market)

Focused Physical Exam

- **Vital signs:** BP, heart rate, temperature
- **Cardiovascular:** irregular rhythm (atrial fibrillation), murmurs
- **Neurologic:** focal neurologic deficits (motor or sensory, usually in one distribution; visual disturbances), impaired speech

Evaluation

- **Labs:**
  - CBC, PT/PTT, Chem 7, lipid panel, ESR.
  - Consider VDRL, antiphospholipid antibodies, thrombophilia workup if indicated (usually young patients, those without risk factors).

- **ECG**

- **Imaging:**
  - **Carotid Doppler U/S** to rule out carotid stenosis for any patient with suspected ischemic cerebrovascular disease
  - **2-D echocardiogram (with bubble study)** to look for left atrial thrombus or mural thrombus in patients with atrial fibrillation or left ventricular systolic dysfunction
  - **Head CT scan or MRI** (diffusion-weighted images) to rule out stroke or hemorrhage

Management

Transient Ischemic Attack

- The risk of stroke after having a TIA is approximately 10% the first year and 5%/yr after.

- Antiplatelet treatment is indicated for secondary prevention of TIAs and stroke.

  - ASA, 75–325 mg PO qd, decreases the risk of stroke by ≥13% and is first-line therapy for secondary prevention of stroke.

  - Clopidogrel (Plavix), 75 mg PO qd, has been shown to decrease the risk of stroke by 8% over ASA (≥21%); however, there were more bleeding complications.

  - Dipyridamole (Persantine), 200 mg PO bid, has a 16% risk reduction of stroke vs placebo.

  - The combination of ASA/dipyridamole (Aggrenox), 1 tablet PO bid, has been shown in one trial to reduce the risk of stroke by 37% vs placebo (ESPS-2).

Carotid Stenosis

- Carotid endarterectomy is indicated for symptomatic patients with >70% carotid artery stenoses. Surgery has also been shown to be beneficial for patients with asymptomatic moderate to severe carotid stenoses (>60%).

- Risk factor modification:

  - Control of HTN and diabetes.

  - Statins (simvastatin [Zocor], 10–40 mg PO qd), may be beneficial in preventing stroke in patients with a history of CAD.

Atrial Fibrillation

- Anticoagulation with warfarin (or ASA if warfarin is contraindicated) is indicated for patients with atrial fibrillation. The risk of stroke is approximately 3–6%/yr.

- Refer to Chap. 8, Cardiology.

When to Refer

- Consider referring to a neurologist patients with multiple TIAs, young patients, and patients in whom the diagnosis is unclear.

- Consider referring to a vascular surgeon or neurosurgeon patients in whom carotid endarterectomy may be indicated.

What to Tell the Patient

- TIAs are "mini-strokes" and are a warning sign that the patient is at high risk for subsequent stroke.

- Risk factor modification is important: good control of diabetes, HTN, and cholesterol can help prevent strokes.

TREMOR

Definition

- Tremor can be divided into three categories: action, resting, and intention tremors.

- Action and resting tremors are common.

- Intention tremors are indicative of cerebellar dysfunction and usually require referral to a neurologist, so they are not discussed here.

Action (Essential, Familial, and Senile)

Differential Diagnosis

- Hyperthyroidism
- Pheochromocytoma
- Wilson's disease
- Medication induced (lithium, amphetamines, amitriptyline)

Key History

- Disappears at rest; asymmetric; can involve hands, head, voice; rarely involves legs; relieved with alcohol ingestion; worsened by anxiety

Key Physical Exam

- Tremor disappears at rest.

Evaluation

- TSH.

- Consider evaluation for pheochromocytoma (plasma-free metanephrines) or Wilson's disease (serum ceruloplasmin level) if indicated.

Management

- Propranolol, 80–240 mg PO qd
- Primidone, 250 mg PO tid

Resting

Differential Diagnosis

- Parkinson's disease
- Medication induced (phenothiazines, haloperidol)
- Shy-Drager syndrome
- Wilson's disease
- Progressive supranuclear palsy

Key History

- Tremor improves with movement. Associated with apathy, emotional lability, social withdrawal, dementia, decreased concentration, slow thought process, depression, sleep disturbances.

Key Physical Exam

- Pill-rolling tremor: 3- to 7-sec cycles, micrographia, autonomic dysfunction, cogwheel rigidity, masked facies, decreased blinking, shuffling gait, postural instability, decreased arm swing

Evaluation

- Consider serum ceruloplasmin to rule out Wilson's disease in patients <40 yrs.

Management

- Mild symptoms:
  - Amantadine, 100 mg PO bid
  - Trihexyphenidyl (Artane), 10 mg PO tid
  - Benztropine (Cogentin), 6 mg PO qd
- Moderate to severe symptoms:
  - L-Dopa/carbidopa (Sinemet), 10/100 mg 1 tablet PO tid; increase to maximum of 1200 mg/day
  - Pergolide, 1 mg PO tid
  - Bromocriptine, 50 mg PO bid
- For very severe symptoms, surgical options are available.
- Physical/occupational, speech therapy can be helpful in maintaining function.
- Tricyclic antidepressants for depressive symptoms.

When to Refer

Refer to a neurologist for more severe cases of Parkinson's or if other causes of resting tremor are suggested.

What to Tell the Patient

- Essential tremor is benign, usually does not progress, and is not associated with Parkinson's disease. It is often familial.

- Symptoms of Parkinson's disease can be controlled with medications. However, despite medical therapy, the disease usually progresses, and there is no curative treatment.

SUGGESTED READING

Diener HC, et al. European Stroke Prevention Study 2 (ESPS-2). *J Neurol Sci* 1996;143:1–13.

Executive Committee for the Asymptomatic Carotid Atherosclerosis Study (ACAS). Endarterectomy for asymptomatic carotid artery stenosis. *JAMA* 1995;273:1421–1428.

Goadsby PJ, Lipton RB, Ferrari MD. Migraine–current understanding and treatment. *N Engl J Med* 2002;346(4):257–270.

Sacco RL, Elkind MS. Update on antiplatelet therapy for stroke prevention. *Arch Intern Med* 2000;160:1579–1582.

Weiner HL, Levitt LP. *Neurology*, 5th ed. Baltimore: Williams & Wilkins, 1994.

18 Ophthalmology

Oh say can you see . . .

CONJUNCTIVITIS, UVEITIS/IRITIS, AND ACUTE ANGLE CLOSURE GLAUCOMA

Red Flags for the Red Eye

- Ocular pain

- Sudden vision loss

- Unilateral red eye associated with nausea/vomiting

- Impaired extraocular movements

- Periorbital swelling

Patients with any red flags should have an ophthalmologic evaluation immediately!

Conjunctivitis

Key History and Physical Exam

- **Allergic:**
  - Often associated with other atopic symptoms (asthma, rhinitis).
  - Symptoms include red eyes, chemosis, watery discharge/tearing.

- **Bacterial** (*Staphylococcus, Streptococcus, Haemophilus, Pseudomonas, Moraxella*). Symptoms include a purulent yellow discharge.

- **Gonococcal:**
  - Acquired through contact with genital secretions.
  - Characterized by abrupt onset of conjunctivitis and copious, thick secretions.

- **Inclusion** (*C. trachomatis*):
  - Found in sexually active persons.
  - Eye findings include discharge, redness, and follicular conjunctivitis with mild keratitis.

- **Viral** (usually adenovirus):
  - Found in association with pharyngitis, fever, preauricular adenopathy.

- Red eye associated with copious watery discharge, often bilateral involvement.

- **Chemical**
  - Caused by exposure to caustic or irritative agent.

Treatment
Allergic

- **Oral antihistamine**
- **Ocular decongestants** (Naphcon-A, 1–2 gtts OU bid–qid)
- **Mast cell stabilizer drops** (olopatadine [Patanol], 2 gtts OU bid)

Bacterial

- **Antibacterial eye drops:** sulfacetamide 10% solution or ointment instilled q8h ×3 days. Bacitracin zinc + polymyxin B sulfate (Polysporin), neomycin + polymyxin B sulfate (Neosporin), ciprofloxacin HCl (Ciloxan), gentamycin, tobramycin, or erythromycin also can be used.

Gonococcal

- **Topical** (bacitracin, erythromycin, or ciprofloxacin) **and systemic antibiotics** (ceftriaxone, 1 g IM ×1).

- Refer immediately to an ophthalmologist to rule out corneal involvement!

Inclusion

- Treat with **doxycycline,** 300 mg PO ×1, then 100 mg PO bid ×14 days.

Viral

- **Treat symptomatically** with cool compresses.

- Can prescribe **antibacterial eye drops** to prevent bacterial superinfection (sulfacetamide 10% solution or ointment instilled q8h ×3 days).

- **Very high level of infectivity.** Limit sharing of towels and wash hands well to limit spread to close contact.

Chemical

- Thoroughly **rinse the eye with water** as soon after the exposure as possible.

- Cool compresses and ocular decongestants (Naphcon-A, 1–2 gtts) are helpful.

- In the case of an acid or alkali injury, copious irrigation and immediate referral to an ophthalmologist are necessary!

Uveitis/Iritis

Key History and Physical Exam

- Symptoms include pain and photophobia.

- Exam reveals pericorneal (ciliary) flush.

- Often associated with systemic illness (Reiter's syndrome, psoriasis, ankylosing spondylitis, Behçet's syndrome, collagen vascular disease, sarcoidosis, toxoplasmosis, TB, syphilis, diabetes, leukemia, inflammatory bowel disease).

- Order screening labs: ANA, rheumatoid factor, ANCA, RPR, UA, Chem 7, CBC, PPD.

Management

- Topical or systemic steroids.

- Rule out HSV or VZV infections before starting steroids—giving steroids with these infections can lead to vision loss!

Acute Angle Closure Glaucoma

Key History and Physical Exam

- Elevated risk in elderly, far-sighted patients, Asians.

- Symptoms include vision loss over minutes to hours, headache, brow and eye pain, and nausea/vomiting.

- Exam findings include red eye, cloudy cornea, mildly dilated pupils that are nonreactive to light, shallow anterior chamber, and increased hardness of eye to palpation.

Management

- **Beta blocker eye drops**, carbonic anhydrase inhibitors (PO or in drop form), pilocarpine, brimonidine ophthalmic (Alphagan), or laser iridectomy.

- Needs *immediate* referral to an ophthalmologist.

When to Refer

Refer any patient with red flag or unresolving symptoms to an ophthalmologist.

OTHER COMMON EYE CONDITIONS

Vision Loss

- **Differential diagnosis:** vitreous hemorrhage, retinal detachment, macular degeneration, TIA, optic neuritis, anterior ischemic optic neuropathy, glaucoma, central retinal artery or vein occlusions. *Any sudden loss of vision requires emergent referral to an ophthalmologist!*

- **Causes of gradual loss of vision:** macular degeneration, chronic glaucoma, diabetic retinopathy, and cataracts. *Refer these to an ophthalmologist on a routine basis.*

- **Legal blindness** is defined as vision that cannot be corrected to better than 20/200.

Hordeolum (Sty)

- *Staphylococcus* abscess of an eyelash follicle.

- Warm, red, and swollen area on the upper or lower lid.

- Treat with warm compresses.

- Bacitracin or erythromycin ointment q3h until resolved. If no improvement in 48 hrs, consider referral to an ophthalmologist for incision and drainage.

Blepharitis

- Inflammation of the eyelid and lashes; may also be associated bacterial infection.

- Strong association with acne rosacea.

- Characterized by burning, itching, and red-rimmed eyelids.

- **Treatment:**

  - Clean eyelids with baby shampoo.

  - Bacitracin or erythromycin ointment daily until resolution.

Herpes Simplex (Dendritic) Keratitis

- Secondary to HSV; may be precipitated by light, immunodeficiency, fever. Patients may have a history of cold sores.

- **Symptoms** include foreign body sensation, eye ache, photophobia.

- **Exam:** Cornea will have a dendritic pattern on slit lamp exam.

- **Treatment**: Viroptic, 1 gtt in the infected eye 5×/day, or acyclovir (Zovirax), 200 mg PO 5×/day.

- These patients should be referred to an ophthalmologist for confirmation of the diagnosis. **Do not prescribe steroid drops—can lead to blindness.**

Corneal Abrasion

- Usually secondary to trauma. Foreign body sensation, mild injection, slit lamp evidence of epithelial disruption (enhanced with fluorescein dye).

- **Treatment** is with Polysporin or erythromycin ointment; refer to ophthalmologist if not better in 24–48 hrs. Do not patch owing to risk of corneal ulcer.

Corneal Ulcer

- Due to infection (most commonly bacterial, but also viral, fungal, and amoebal).

- **Risk factors:** Contact lens wearers and history of corneal abrasion that has been patched.

- **Symptoms:** Foreign body sensation, pain, and blurred vision.

- **Exam:** White area in the cornea (hypopyon).

- **Treatment** is with an antibacterial drop; however, if there is thinning of the cornea, a culture should be obtained before treatment.

- **Stop all contact lens wear until symptoms resolve.**

- **Requires immediate referral to an ophthalmologist.**

Chronic Open Angle Glaucoma

- **Risk factors:** African-Americans, elderly, family history, diabetes.

- **Symptoms:** Gradual loss of peripheral vision over years, halos around lights, tunnel vision.

- **Exam:** Increased cup to disk ratio and increased ocular pressure.

- **Treatment:** Beta blocker eye drops, carbonic anhydrase inhibitor eye drops, latanoprost (Xalatan), Alphagan, or laser trabeculoplasty.

- Needs referral to an ophthalmologist.

Trauma

- Refer immediately to an ophthalmologist.

Eye Findings in Systemic Illnesses

- An eye exam may give evidence of the severity and chronicity of other medical conditions, such as HTN, diabetes, sickle cell anemia, HIV, and Graves' disease. These patients should be referred to an opthalmologist for evaluation.

- **Diabetes:**

  - Nonproliferative (microaneurysms, hemorrhages, hard exudates) and proliferative retinopathy (neovascularization that can be complicated by vitreous hemorrhage and/or retinal detachment).

  - **Yearly exams** are recommended for type I diabetics beginning 3–5 yrs after diagnosis and starting immediately for type II diabetics.

- **HTN:**
  - Acute elevated BP (accelerated HTN) leads to retinopathy (hemorrhages/exudates).
  - Findings in malignant HTN include retinopathy and papilledema.
  - Chronic HTN results in arterial narrowing, arteriovenous nicking, and copper wiring.
- **Sickle cell anemia:** Proliferative retinopathy.
- **AIDS:** Hemorrhages, exudates, microaneurysm, CMV retinitis, fungal endophthalmitis, HSV/VZV, and Kaposi's sarcoma.
- **Graves' disease:** Exophthalmos and diplopia.

When to Refer

Immediately refer to an ophthalmologist any patients with:

- Sudden loss of vision
- Ocular trauma
- Orbital cellulitis
- Gonococcal conjunctivitis
- Herpes simplex keratitis
- Acute angle closure glaucoma
- Central retinal artery/vein occlusion
- Any red eye that fails to resolve
- Any red flags

What to Tell the Patient

- Any vision symptoms should be taken seriously and evaluated by a physician.
- Diabetic patients should have their eyes examined yearly, as diabetic retinopathy can lead to vision loss.
- African-Americans, older individuals, and those with a family history are at increased risk for glaucoma and should be evaluated by an ophthalmologist q3–5yrs with tonometric evaluation.

SUGGESTED READING

Liebowitz HM. The red eye. *N Engl J Med* 2000;343(5):345–351.
Vaughan DG, Asbury T, Riordan-Eva P. *General ophthalmology,* 14th ed. New York: Appleton & Lange, 1995.

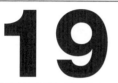

Orthopedics

Sticks and stones may break my bones, but clinic will never hurt me...

ANKLE AND FOOT PAIN
Differential Diagnosis

- **Ankle pain:** ligamentous injury (sprain, tear), tendon injury, ankle fracture, ankle dislocation
- **Foot pain:** puncture/blunt trauma, foot/toe fracture, ligamentous injury, tendon injury, plantar fasciitis

Key History
Orthopedic

- Mechanism of injury, injury circumstances (associated injuries?)
- Direction/position of applied force (inversion [lateral structure injury], eversion [medial injury])
- Any sounds associated with injury ("pop" [ligament injury]; "crack" [fracture])
- Time of injury/pain (acute, chronic)
- Puncture wound (possible foreign bodies, infection)
- Associated fall (trip/slip, syncope, substance abuse)
- Palliative/provoking factors (pain with first step in the morning, first few steps of running [plantar fasciitis])
- Overuse injury (joggers, occupation requiring standing [plantar fasciitis])

Medical History

- Chronic conditions (diabetes mellitus, peripheral vascular disease, neurologic deficiency), previous trauma
- Tetanus vaccination status

Medications
- Steroids (may mask swelling)
- NSAID use

Social History
- Alcohol or drug abuse (withdrawal)
- Smoking (impaired wound healing)

Focused Physical Exam

- **General:** Overall degree of discomfort.

- **Ankle and foot:**

  - Abnormal **foot biomechanics** (pes planus, pes cavus, discordant leg length).

  - **Inspection** for appearance (color/bruising, swelling, hematoma, position, skin).

  - **Palpate,** starting away from affected area (crepitus, point tenderness).

  - Passive/active **range of motion** of each joint.

  - **Ankle anterior drawer test:** With leg hanging over side of bed, hold heel of foot in one hand, distal leg in other; pull heel anteriorly. Positive if >2 mm movement vs other ankle (displacement of foot anteriorly on tibia).

  - **Talar tilt test:** Evert/invert foot: >10-degree difference vs opposite foot is positive (inversion suggests injury to >2 lateral collateral ligaments; eversion suggests deltoid compromise).

  - **Thompson test:** With patient prone, squeeze midcalf. Should induce plantar flexion if Achilles tendon intact.

  - **Suspected plantar fasciitis:** Confirm with reproducible tenderness on palpation of plantar fascia; worse with dorsiflexion of the toes.

- **Wound:** Evidence of foreign body, debris.

- **Knee:** Palpate, range of motion.

- **Vascular:** Assess peripheral pulses; compare vs contralateral side (dorsalis pedis, posterior tibialis, capillary refill).

- **Neurologic:** Motor strength and sensation, orientation/alertness, ability to ambulate on injury.

Evaluation

X-Ray

- **Standard ankle films:**

  - Anteroposterior, lateral, mortise (joint) views.

  - Should include base of fifth metatarsal.

  - Look for widening of the ankle mortise (indication for referral to an orthopedic surgeon).

  - **Soft tissue penetration:** Useful in evaluating for presence of possible foreign object.

TABLE 19-1.
OTTAWA ANKLE RULES[a,b]

Ankle radiographs necessary:

Pain near malleoli *and*

Unable to weight bear >4 steps immediately and in office/ED *or*

Bony tenderness over posterior edge/tip of either malleolus

Foot radiographs necessary:

Pain in midfoot *and*

Bone tenderness at navicular, cuboid, or base fifth metatarsal

[a]These are only guidelines.
[b]**Always order x-rays in the following situations:** intoxication, pediatric cases, neurologic deficit/head injury, and if there are multiple associated injuries.

- Use **Ottawa rules** (Table 19-1) as guide for when to order x-rays (increase diagnostic yield).

CT, MRI, and Stress Views

Limited value in initial evaluation (reserve for specialist).

Management

- **A pulseless foot is a medical emergency in the setting of dislocation or displaced fracture!** *Do not wait for x-rays to initiate intervention.* Seek immediate orthopedic assistance; if unavailable, consider realigning foot by stabilizing leg and restoring foot to neutral position (hang leg over side of bed, apply downward traction to heel/foot, slide into realignment, recheck for pulse).

- The **initial goal** in the clinic with any ankle or foot injury is to stabilize the foot or ankle to prevent further injury. Place foot/ankle in neutral position using pillow, roll splint, or air cast; then transport to the ED.

Pain Relief

- Ibuprofen, 400–800 mg PO tid (take with meals to decrease GI side effects)

- Naproxen, 250–500 mg PO bid

- Acetaminophen (APAP), 500–1000 mg PO tid–qid (max of 4 g/day total APAP if normal liver function)

- APAP with codeine (Tylenol #3), 500 mg/30 mg, 1–2 tabs PO tid prn for severe pain

- APAP with oxycodone (Percocet), 500 mg/7.5 mg, 1 tab PO qid prn for very severe pain

Ankle Fractures

Require transfer to ED after stabilization for reduction and/or casting.

Stable Ankle Sprains

- "RICE-N": rest, ice (20 mins q4h), compression dressing (elastic bandage), elevation (1–2 days of extremity elevation); NSAIDs (see page 213).

- Weight bear as tolerated in 48–72 hrs. Add exercise in 4–5 days.

- Avoid hot water baths (may actually worsen swelling in first few days).

- Consider immobilization with a cast or leg orthotic if early mobilization is required.

- Long-term treatment includes protective taping or bracing for exercise and strengthening exercises.

- Pain may persist for weeks, particularly with "high ankle" sprain (damage to the tibiofibular syndesmosis). If symptoms do not resolve, consider repeating x-rays and referring to orthopedic surgeon for further evaluation and management.

Toe Dislocations

Second to fifth toes easily reduced with traction, forced dorsiflexion, and then reduction with plantar flexion.

Toe Fractures

Immobilize if nondisplaced second to fourth toe with "buddy taping"; use flat orthopedic shoe.

Plantar Fasciitis

- Generally self-limiting (but may last up to 18 mos).

- Rest with substitution of lower-intensity/weight-bearing activity.

- Stretches/strengthening (curb stretches, rolling stretches over a tennis ball, toe-taps).

- Proper-fitting tennis shoes, orthotics if any biomechanical abnormalities, night splints.

- Antiinflammatory: NSAIDs (see page 213), ice (20 mins/day after activity).

- Corticosteroid injections: to be performed by an experienced person in refractory cases.

- Surgery (plantar fasciotomy) is reserved for cases unresponsive to the above interventions.

When to Refer

- At follow-up, if not substantially improved or worse, consider referral.

- *Immediately* with neurovascular compromise.

- Any fracture or dislocation (other than nondisplaced toe fracture or second to fifth toe dislocation).

- Joint instability or inability to ambulate.

- Injuries that fail to improve with conservative management.

- *Any* injury that you are unsure how to manage.

What to Tell the Patient

- Most ankle sprains heal well regardless of grade, and primary surgical repair offers little advantage over conservative management.

- Should surgery become necessary because of sprain after several weeks of persistent pain, delayed surgery can be performed without sacrifice of outcome.

- "Heel spurs" (bony osteophytes) on x-ray are **not** pathologic: 15–25% of asymptomatic individuals have them, and often those with plantar fasciitis do not.

LOW BACK PAIN
Etiology
Acute

- Low back spasm/strain

- Disk herniation

- Fracture (compression, trauma, pathologic)

- Infection (osteomyelitis, epidural abscess)

- Referred pain (renal, aortic, GI, genitourinary, hip)

- Malignancy (primary, metastatic)

Chronic

- Degenerative joint/disk disease

- Spinal stenosis

- Rheumatic disease (seronegative spondyloarthropathy)

- Spondylolisthesis/spondylosis

- Malignancy

Key History

- **General:** Age (younger: spasm/strain, seronegative spondyloarthropathy; older: malignancy, spinal stenosis), weight loss, fever, chills, sweats

- **Orthopedic:**
  - Characterize pain: sharp, dull, achy
  - Pain intensity, location, radiation
  - Pain onset: sudden (spasm, strain, fracture, herniation, referred pain, infection), gradual (malignancy, degenerative joint disease [DJD], seronegative spondyloarthropathy)
  - Timing: worse in morning (seronegative spondyloarthropathy), worse with exertion (spasm, strain, DJD)
  - Associated events: fall (fracture, spasm, strain), sports/lifting (spasm/strain, pathologic injury)
  - Palliative factors: rest (DJD, spasm, strain), exercise (seronegative spondyloarthropathy)

- **Medical history:** malignancy, infection (endocarditis), osteoporosis, immunocompromised, chronic infection (genitourinary, pulmonary, skin), prior disk disease

- **Social history:** IV drug use (abscess), substance abuse (accident risk), secondary gain issues

Red Flags for Back Pain

General

- Severe nighttime pain
- Pain worse at rest
- Pain worse in supine position
- Weight loss, fever, chills
- Failure of conservative treatment

Cauda Equina Syndrome

- Saddle anesthesia
- New-onset bowel/bladder dysfunction
- Progressive lower extremity neurologic deficit
- Perianal/perineal sensory loss, anal sphincter laxity

Tumor/Infection

- Age <20 or >50
- History of malignancy

- History of chronic infection
- Immunosuppression (steroids, HIV positive)
- History of IV drug use
- Weight loss, fevers, chills, sweats

Fracture

- Major trauma (serious fall, motor vehicle accident)
- Minor trauma (with osteoporosis/elderly)

Focused Physical Exam

- **General:** weight (obese, weight loss), appearance (chronically ill, septic)

- **Back:** asymmetry, erythema, warmth, masses, range of motion, point tenderness (lumbar, sacroiliac joint)

  - *Shober test*: With patient standing, mark skin at L5 and make another mark 10 cm above this point; have patient bend forward and measure distance between points (<4 cm = decreased lumbar flexion). Positive tests are concerning for seronegative spondyloarthropathy.

  - *Straight leg test*: While supine, raise and straighten patient's relaxed leg until pain occurs (dorsiflexion may worsen pain); positive if radicular pain in nerve distribution ("crossed straight leg" positive if raising leg causes contralateral radicular pain).

  - *Waddell signs*: Discordant sitting/supine straight leg raise, severe pain with light touch, nondermatomal sensory/motor complaints, pain with axial loading by pressing down on patient's skull (suggestive of "supratentorial" component to pain).

- **Neurologic:** motor strength, reflexes, sensory loss in nerve root distribution (Table 19-2)

Evaluation and Management

- See **Table 19-3 for evaluation and treatment of** specific **common etiologies.**

- **Assess for red flags** and consider possible sources of referred pain. If no red flags and referred pain is unlikely, treat presumptive cause conservatively and reassess in 2–4 wks:

  - Acetaminophen, 500–1000 mg PO tid, or ibuprofen, 400–800 mg PO tid.

  - Stretching exercises/walking or physical therapy.

- If red flags present, initiate further workup as indicated, starting with lumbosacral spine films, and consider specialist referral as appropriate.

TABLE 19-2.
LOW BACK PAIN: NERVE ROOT DISTRIBUTION

Nerve root	L4	L5	S1
Pain	Hip, anterolateral thigh	Gluteal, lateral thigh to ankle	Gluteal, posterolateral thigh to ankle
Numbness	Inner thigh to knee	Lateral calf	Posterior calf, posterolateral foot
Motor weakness	Quadriceps extension	Dorsiflexion foot/great toe	Plantar flexion foot/great toe
Screening test	Weak squat/rise	Heel ambulation	Toe ambulation
Reflexes diminished	Knee jerk	—	Ankle jerk

- **If tumor/infection red flags present:** Check ESR, CBC, UA; consider MRI or bone scan if unrevealing.
- **If cauda equina red flags present:** MRI and neurosurgical consult *immediately.*
- **At 2- to 4-wk reassessment:**
  - If improved pain and increased activity tolerance, continue or titrate down treatment.
  - If no improvement or new neurologic symptoms after 4 wks, reassess for red flags.
  - If no red flags, consider advancing symptomatic treatment (add or increase pain medication, add muscle relaxant).
  - If red flags are present, consider further imaging/evaluation as above and consider appropriate referrals if indicated.
- If, by **8–12 wks,** patient is still without improvement, consider referral to orthopedic surgeon or sports medicine specialist.

What to Tell the Patient

- 9 of 10 patients with low back pain will recover fully by 8–12 wks with conservative management.
- Routine use of expensive imaging (CT/MRI) is **not** indicated, as abnormal findings are not specific (1 of 4 healthy persons has herniated disk on CT).
- Bed rest >2 days has been shown to be more harmful than beneficial.
- **Surgery is not necessarily better than conservative therapy.** Initial response to surgery, when indicated, is approximately 90% at 1 yr, but by 4 yrs the improvement is equal to conservative management (60% improvement).

TABLE 19-3.
EVALUATION AND TREATMENT OF SPECIFIC LOW BACK PAIN ETIOLOGIES

Back pain etiology	Historical clues	Physical exam	Specific evaluation	Management
Low back sprain/strain	No red flags	No red flags Point tenderness over musculoligamentous structures	No specific evaluation indicated for 4 wks	Conservative therapy with analgesics and physical therapy
Compression fracture	Acute/severe pain, possibly after trauma/lifting Age >50 (especially >70)	Spinal percussion tenderness (thoracic/upper lumbar)	L/S spine films (30–40% loss of height needed to detect) DEXA scan Consider possibility of pathologic fracture	Analgesics (including narcotics acutely) Osteoporosis management (see Chap. 10, Endocrinology)
Cauda equina syndrome (spinal cord compression)	Cauda equina red flags (saddle anesthesia, bladder/bowel dysfunction) History of malignancy (prostate, breast, lung, renal, GI, thyroid, multiple myeloma, lymphoma)	Cauda equina red flags (loss of rectal tone, LE neurologic deficit in nerve root distributions) Ambulation (if unable to ambulate, prognosis poor)	Stat MRI at affected level Postvoid residuals (urinary retention >100 cc)	*Consult neurosurgery immediately* and consider starting high-dose dexamethasone (10 mg IV q6h)

(continued)

TABLE 19-3.
CONTINUED

220

Back pain etiology	Historical clues	Physical exam	Specific evaluation	Management
Lumbar disk herniation (protrusion of nucleus pulposus thru annulus fibrosis)	Pain worse with sitting, straining, cough Sciatica (radiating pain down posterior leg) History of previous back pain	Impaired nerve root function (see Table 19-2) Positive straight leg test	L/S spine films (evaluate for other pathology) MRI (confirmatory test, positive in 20–30% of asymptomatic patients)	Conservative if no red flags; 80% improve in 6 wks Surgery (severe/progressive neurologic deficits, cauda equina syndrome)
Spinal stenosis (narrowing of root canal, lumbar spinal canal, or intervertebral foramen)	Nonspecific back pain (usually stable over time) "Pseudoclaudication": buttock/thigh burning/cramping with spinal extension (standing, walking uphill); relief with sitting/lying Acquired (Paget's, hyperparathyroid, Cushing's, acromegaly)	Straight leg test (usually negative) Usually nonspecific; may have subtle abnormalities	L/S spine films (degenerative disk or vertebral changes) CT or MRI (confirmatory test, positive in 20% of asymptomatic patients)	Conservative medical therapy: analgesics, NSAIDs, exercise, weight loss Surgery (lumbar laminectomy) for refractory symptoms

| Seronegative spondyloarthropathy (ankylosing spondylitis, Reiter's disease, psoriatic arthritis, inflammatory bowel disease) | M>F (3:1), begins in teens–20s

Insidious onset, persistent (>90 days), bilateral, morning stiffness, improves with exercise

Preceding GI illness, urethritis (Reiter's) | Enthesitis (inflammation of osseous attachments of ligaments/tendons)

Shober's test positive

Kyphosis

Urethritis, uveitis (Reiter's)

Shoulder/hip involvement | L/S spine films: "bamboo spine": squaring of vertebral bodies with intervertebral disk ossification

SI joint films: subchondral blurring, erosions, sclerosis

Lab tests: elevated ESR, normochromic anemia, elevated IgA, HLA-B27 positive | Early exercise/PT essential in slowing progression

NSAIDs for pain/stiffness

Consider methotrexate, sulfasalazine, steroids, immunosuppressants

Corticosteroid injections for enthesitis, SI joint, peripheral arthritis

Surgery for severe hip, C spine, kyphosis (wedge resection) |

LE, lower extremity; L/S, lumbosacral; PT, physical therapy; SI, sacroiliac.

GOUT
Definition
Attacks of arthritis caused by urate deposition.

Differential Diagnosis

- Pseudogout (calcium pyrophosphate deposition disease)
- Reiter's syndrome (enthesopathy)
- Reactive arthritis, rheumatoid arthritis (RA), psoriatic arthritis, infectious arthritis

Key History

- **General:** fever, chills (infection)
- **Orthopedic:**
  - Sudden onset of severe pain
  - Pain that awoke patient from sleep
  - Light touch painful (gout)
  - Number of joints involved (monoarticular = gout, septic arthritis; polyarticular = systemic arthritis)
  - Location of pain (commonly first metatarsophalangeal [MTP] joint for gout)
  - Gout triggers (alcohol binge, dehydration, recent surgery, illness, trauma)
- **Medical history:** history of previous gout attacks, renal disease (decreased urate clearance), diabetes insipidus, diabetes mellitus, hyperlipidemia, hypothyroidism, HTN (diuretic use), psoriasis (psoriatic arthritis), atherosclerosis, elevated parathyroid hormone (pseudogout), malignancy (tumor lysis syndrome with leukemia, lymphoma)
- **Medications:** salicylates, thiazide/loop diuretics, pyrazinamide, ethambutol, cyclosporine, heparin
- **Social history:** diet (meats, organ foods [e.g., liver], seafood, yeasts/breads, beans), alcohol consumption, activity (increased exercise)

Focused Physical Exam

- **Vital signs:** fever (infection)
- **General:** obesity, gender (male, postmenopausal female), age (40–60)
- **HEENT:** tophi on ears

- **Orthopedic:**
  - Red, swollen joint; exquisitely painful to light touch
  - Joints commonly involved in gout: first MTP ("podagra"), ankle, foot, knee, elbow, finger
  - Symmetric joint involvement (RA)
- **Skin:** rashes (psoriasis)

Evaluation

- **Joint aspiration** to evaluate for crystals:
  - Send aspirate for **gram stain** and **culture** (rule out septic arthritis) and **leukocyte count with differential** (10,000–100,000 with 50–90% polymorphonuclear neutrophils suggestive of inflammatory arthritis).
  - Can also do **tophi aspiration** to look for urate crystals.
  - **Needle-shaped, negatively birefringent crystals** in gout vs **rhomboid-shaped, positively birefringent crystals** (pseudogout).
- **Serum uric acid:**
  - Draw after acute attack has resolved.
  - May be high (>8 mg/dL in men; >7 mg/dL in women) or normal.
- **Labs:** Check Chem 7, Mg, Ca, CBC, and TSH.
- **Urine:**
  - 24-hr urine for uric acid after symptoms of acute attack resolved.
  - >800 mg/day is indicative of overproduction; <800 mg/day is indicative of underexcretion.
- **Joint x-ray:**
  - Not routinely indicated
  - Normal early with gout
  - Evidence of joint destruction with advanced gout or other arthritis (e.g., rheumatoid, psoriatic)
  - Chondrocalcinosis (pseudogout)

Management
Acute Attack

- Without treatment, gout attacks generally last 7–10 days. However, treatment can shorten the duration of attacks.

- **Symptomatic treatment** includes bed rest and warm soaks.

- **Pharmacologic options:**

  - **NSAIDs:** indomethacin, 50–100 mg PO tid; wean over 1 wk as attack wanes. Use with caution in renal dysfunction and with history of GI bleed or peptic ulcer disease.

  - **Other NSAIDs** (also wean over 1 wk): ibuprofen, 400–800 mg PO tid; naproxen, 250–500 mg PO tid.

  - **Colchicine,** 1–2 mg PO ×1, then 0.5 mg PO q2h until total of 8 mg given or abdominal pain, nausea/vomiting, or diarrhea. Avoid in renal/hepatic dysfunction; also small risk of agranulocytosis, aplastic anemia, peripheral neuritis.

  - **Corticosteroids:** methylprednisolone (Medrol), 5–60 mg intraarticular (depending on joint size), or prednisone, 20–40 mg PO qd, tapering over 7–10 days. Use only if colchicines/NSAIDs contraindicated.

  - **Rule out infection before giving steroids.**

Prophylaxis

- Indicated in patients with a high uric acid level. Stop after uric acid level has normalized. Colchicine, 0.5–0.6 mg PO qd–bid ×12 wks, or indomethacin, 50–100 mg PO qd ×8–12 wks, can be used.

Hyperuricemia

- Asymptomatic hyperuricemia does not need to be treated, as many patients never develop gout.

  - Use **uricosuric drugs** to increase renal urate excretion in underexcreters.

    - **Probenecid,** 0.5 mg PO bid–tid. Side effects: headache, dizziness, nausea, vomiting. Contraindicated in G6PD deficiency.

    - **Sulfinpyrazone:** Start at 100–200 mg PO bid ×1 wk, then increase to maintenance dose (max. 400 mg PO bid). Side effects: nausea, dyspepsia, rash, aplastic anemia, agranulocytosis, thrombocytopenia.

    - Add $NaHCO_3$, 1 g PO tid for 2–3 wks, to minimize risk of urolithiasis.

  - Use **xanthine oxidase inhibitors** to decrease urate synthesis in patients with elevated urate production or decreased urate clearance (CrCl <60 mL/min).

    - **Allopurinol,** 50–100 mg PO qd, titrate up to 100–300 mg PO qd over 3–4 wks. Use lowest dose possible to keep serum urate <6 mg/dL. Side effects: rash, elevated LFTs, nausea, pruritus. **Contraindicated** in renal failure or concurrent 6-MP or azathioprine.

- Delay use until several weeks after gout attack to minimize risk of precipitating gout attack (can also give with concomitant colchicine).

What to Tell the Patient

- Weight loss and control of BP and other medical conditions may decrease frequency of attacks.

- Limit alcohol, particularly beer.

- Dietary modifications: avoidance of high-purine foods (meats, sardines, seafood, legumes, anchovies, sweetbreads).

- Encourage regular increased oral fluid intake, as dehydration may precipitate attacks.

- Avoid tight shoes; they may cause joint stress and precipitate attack.

- Let physician know if medications are poorly tolerated; stopping them may lead to return of gout.

- Approximately 75% of patients have a recurrent attack within 2 yrs of the first attack.

KNEE PAIN
Differential Diagnosis

See Table 19-4.

Key History

- **General:** fever, chills, sweats (septic joint)
- **Orthopedic:** See Table 19-4.
- **Medical history:**
  - Knee injuries/disorders/surgery (when/how injury occurred, treatments received)
  - STDs/gonorrhea (septic arthritis)
  - Overlying infection/abrasion
  - Immunocompromised (HIV, steroids, diabetes mellitus)
- **Medications:** NSAIDs, narcotics, APAP usage
- **Social history:** any recent change in footwear, change in activity (increased frequency/intensity), history of IV drug use

TABLE 19-4.
EVALUATION AND TREATMENT OF COMMON
KNEE INJURIES

Injury	History	Exam findings	Further testing/treatment
Meniscal tear	Recent/previous twisting/squatting injury (especially with weight bearing)	Tenderness to palpation at joint line	X-rays normal; MRI can confirm meniscal injury
	"Clicks" or "locking" of knee	Positive McMurray's/Apley's test	Symptomatic management ("RICE-N," ROM exercises)
	Rotational pain	Inability to squat	Arthroscopic evaluation/repair
Collateral ligament tear (ACL, PCL, MCL, LCL)	Acute injury in which "joint gave out"; inability to continue activity; "pop" felt/heard	Effusions/swelling	X-rays normal; MRI to confirm ligament tear/evaluate for concurrent meniscus injury
ACL	Cut/pivot or hyperextension injury, valgus force to knee rotated externally	Positive anterior drawer/Lachman's	Symptomatic management ("RICE-N," ROM exercises)
PCL	Blow to tibia anteriorly (dashboard in motor vehicle accident)	Posterior drawer	Referral to specialist for possible surgical repair
LCL	Varus force	Lateral tenderness, ipsilateral laxity, "joint opening"	
MCL	Valgus force	Medial tenderness, ipsilateral laxity, "joint opening"	
Ligamentous sprain (ACL, PCL, MCL, LCL)	Similar mechanism of injury as above	Grade 1: pain, mild disability	X-rays normal Symptomatic management ("RICE-N," ROM exercises)
		Grade 2: pain, moderate disability, laxity with crisp end point	

(*continued*)

TABLE 19-4.
CONTINUED

Injury	History	Exam findings	Further testing/ treatment
		Grade 3: complete rupture with instability (see above)	
Septic arthritis	Fevers, chills, sweats; progressive course over hrs–days; no history of trauma/injury	Joint warmth/ erythema	Joint aspiration: Gram stain with PMNs/organisms + culture
	History of superficial infection overlying joint	Absence of ligamentous/meniscal abnormalities	CBC: leukocytosis
	History of previous gonococcal infection/STDs	Exquisitely painful to move	Hospitalization for repeated aspiration/surgical débridement and IV antibiotics necessary
	History of IV drug use		
	History of previous injury, surgery (especially with hardware)		
	Immunocompromised		
Patellar dislocation	History of direct blow to knee or external rotational force	Frequently spontaneously reduces before presentation	X-ray (AP/lateral): lateral deviation of patella, assess for osteochondral fracture (may require arthroscopic surgery)
		Patellar apprehension test	
Hemarthrosis	History of recent trauma, ligamentous or meniscal injury, or bleeding disorder (hemophilia)	Assess for effusion, ligament stability (above), or fracture (below)	Joint aspiration: pink, red, or brown fluid
			X-ray: assess for fracture
Overuse syndrome	Repetitive recreational excess ("weekend warrior") or occupational movement	Paucity of objective findings; ligament/ meniscal exams unrevealing	No further imaging indicated
	Progressive course over several days/ wks		Conservative management ("RICE-N," support brace for comfort)

(continued)

TABLE 19-4.
CONTINUED

Injury	History	Exam findings	Further testing/ treatment
Osteoarthritis	History of trauma Pain with use, relief with rest Chronic, progressive course	Crepitus, joint hyperthrophy; may be normal	Knee x-rays: osteophytes, joint space narrowing See "Osteoarthritis"
Rheumatoid arthritis	Insidious onset, morning stiffness, fatigue Multiple joints involved (MCP, PIP, wrist)	Joint warmth, erythema, tenderness; symmetric involvement of joints; decreased ROM	Knee x-rays: subchondral cysts, marginal erosions, osteopenia Labs: rheumatoid factor Rx: NSAIDs, DMARDs (e.g., methotrexate)
Crystalline arthropathy (gout, pseudogout)	Acute-onset, severe joint pain Multiple joints involved in past (unusual to have knee as herald joint)	Joint warmth, erythema, tenderness	Knee x-rays: normal or chondrocalcinosis ("pseudogout") Arthrocentesis: urate (negative birefringent needles) or Ca pyrophosphate (positive birefringent rhomboid crystals)

ACL, anterior collateral ligament; AP, anteroposterior; DMARD, disease-modifying antirheumatic drugs; LCL, lateral collateral ligament; MCL, medial collateral ligament; MCP, metacarpophalangeal; MVA, motor vehicle accident; PCL, posterior collateral ligament; PIP, proximal interphalangeal; PMN, polymorphonuclear neutrophil; ROM, range of motion.

Focused Physical Exam

- Assess knee with radiographs before extensive manipulation if considering possible fracture.
- **General:** overall level of discomfort (may need to give analgesics or attempt to repeat exam in 24 hrs if severe pain).
- **Knee:**
  - Always compare findings to contralateral side.

- **Inspection:** observe standing, walking, and squatting; look for symmetry, swelling, effusions, ecchymoses.

- **Palpate** (supine, knee flexed to 90 degrees): begin distal from injury and assess for swelling in joint and soft tissue; check collateral ligaments and patella and look for effusions ("ballotable" patella).

- **Measure** knee for swelling and thigh and calf for atrophy (occurs 2–3 wks after injury without aggressive therapy).

- **Range of motion:** active and passive (should have 0–15 degrees extension, 135 degrees flexion).

- **Neurologic:** motor function/strength, sensation.

- **Vascular:** pulses (popliteal, dorsalis pedis, posterior tibialis).

- **Special tests:**

  - **Drawer test** (anterior collateral ligament [ACL]/posterior collateral ligament [PCL]): With patient supine, have patient bend knee to 90 degrees; cup hand behind calf and draw tibia forward to feel for "crisp" end point (ACL); push tibia back to assess PCL end point for "crispness."

  - **Lachman's test** (ACL/PCL): Similar to drawer test (done with patient supine). Leg bend to 15–30 degrees; hold distal femur in one hand, proximal tibia in the other, and assess for "crisp" end points.

  - **Collateral ligaments** (lateral collateral ligament [LCL]/medial collateral ligament [MCL]): Hold lower leg and apply valgus and varus stresses in full extension and with the knee at 30 degrees; look for pain/laxity of the knee.

  - **McMurray's test** (meniscal tear): With knee fully flexed, gradually extend to 90 degrees, holding first in full internal rotation (lateral meniscus) and then in full external rotation (medial meniscus); pain or "click" may signify meniscal injury.

  - **Apley's compression test** (meniscal tear): With patient prone and knee flexed to 90 degrees, apply axial compressive load while exerting medial and then lateral rotation; assess for medial/lateral pain suggestive of possible meniscal injury.

  - **Patellar apprehension test** (patellar dislocation): Push patella laterally with knee flexed to 30 degrees; produces discomfort.

Evaluation

- See Table 19-4 for details on specific injuries.

TABLE 19-5.
GENERAL INDICATIONS FOR X-RAYS WITH KNEE PAIN

Age >55, especially if history of malignancy

Tenderness at head of fibula

Isolated patellar tenderness

Inability to flex knee to 90 degrees

Inability to bear weight

Inability to walk several steps

Inability to transfer weight to both legs

Effusion/ecchymosis present

- **Standard knee x-rays:** See Table 19-5 for indications.
- **MRI/CT:** Reserve for specialist to order appropriate study.
- **Labs:** Consider CBC (infection or fracture), serum urate (gout), rheumatoid factor (RF), and type and cross (fracture).
- **Blood cultures** (infection): special cultures needed for *Neisseria gonorrhea* (also consider vaginal/urethral swabs).
- **Joint aspiration:** cell count, Gram stain/culture (infection), crystals. See Chap. 25, Procedures.

Management

- **"RICE-N":** **r**est, **i**ce (20 mins q4h), **c**ompression dressing (elastic bandage), **e**levation (1–2 days of extremity elevation); **N**SAIDs (see below), crutch ambulation without weight bearing for 48 hrs.
- **Pain control/antiinflammatory agents:**
  - Ibuprofen, 200–800 mg PO tid scheduled.
  - Naproxen, 250–500 mg PO bid scheduled.
  - APAP, 500 mg 1–2 tablets PO q6–8h scheduled (not to exceed total of 3–4 g/day in patient without alcohol use and normal liver function).
  - APAP with codeine (Tylenol #3), 500 mg/30 mg 1–2 tablets PO q6h for short-term, severe pain.
  - APAP with oxycodone (Percocet), 500 mg/7.5 mg 1 tablet PO qid prn for very severe pain.
- See Table 19-4 for management of specific conditions.

When to Refer

- **Immediately** if evidence of knee dislocation or vascular/neurologic compromise

- Evidence of fracture or meniscal or ligamentous tear

- Septic arthritis for surgical drainage and débridement

- Injuries that fail to improve with conservative management

- Any injury that you are unsure how to manage

OSTEOARTHRITIS (OA)
Key History

- **Orthopedic:**

  - Location of joint pain

  - Stiffness (briefly in a.m.)

  - Swelling

  - Loss of function (poor grip, difficulty with grooming or ambulation)

  - Number of joints

  - Exacerbating/relieving factors (exacerbated by weight bearing, movement, activity; relieved by rest)

  - Sudden, acute pain (fracture or collapse of an avascular bone segment)

- **Medical history:** obesity, joint dysplasia (developmental hip displacement), trauma, past joint surgeries, RA

- **Family history:** RA, OA

- **Social history:** occupation (bending, heavy lifting, operating heavy machinery), hobbies, athletic activities

Focused Physical Exam

- **General:** weight, BMI (obesity)

- **Musculoskeletal:** mild tenderness to palpation, bony enlargement, crepitus, range of motion, gait (limping or stiff), limb asymmetry, mild inflammation, erythema, effusion, muscle wasting (long-standing OA), stability of joint (usually no instability present in OA)

- Notable for lack of signs of acute synovitis (e.g., warmth, redness)

Evaluation

- **Labs:** no specific labs. Consider drawing rheumatoid factor, ANA, ENA, ESR to rule out collagen vascular diseases (if indicated).

- **Joint x-rays:** asymmetric narrowing of joint space, subchondral sclerosis bone, subchondral cysts, osteophytes, and bone remodeling.

- **Joint aspiration:** not routinely indicated for OA, performed to rule out other causes of joint inflammation.

Management

- **OA has no cure,** so treatment centers upon pain control and improving quality of life.

- **Nonpharmacologic therapy** is an important part of treating OA:

  - **Weight loss.**

  - An **exercise program** can improve mobility and function as well as decrease pain and halt succession of symptoms. Range of motion and flexibility exercises, cardiovascular exercise, and muscle conditioning (especially quadriceps strengthening) are all helpful.

  - **Walkers or canes** for support.

  - **Bracing and corrective footwear** (shock-absorbing footwear, heel wedging, support sleeves, dynamic bracing, and taping) can be used to relieve knee OA.

  - **Physical and occupational therapy** are beneficial to increase range of motion and strength, especially in patients with functional limitations due to OA.

- **Medications** are indicated for pain control:

  - **APAP** is first-line therapy for mild to moderate pain. Start at 325–1000 mg PO q6h, max. 4 g/day (caution in patients with a history of liver disease, alcohol abuse, and warfarin use [prolongs half-life]).

  - **NSAIDS** can be used in patients who don't respond to APAP.

    - **Nonselective NSAIDs** (e.g., ibuprofen, 600 mg PO q6–8h) or **COX-2–specific inhibitors** (rofecoxib [Vioxx], 25–50 mg PO qd, or celecoxib [Celebrex], 100–200 mg PO bid) have been shown to be equally effective in reducing joint pain.

    - **COX-2–specific inhibitor or a nonselective NSAID + gastroprotective therapy** (misoprostol [Cytotec], 200 µg PO qid, omeprazole [Prilosec], or high-dose H_2-blockers) should be used in patients at high risk of GI events (see below).

- Use with caution in patients at risk for GI bleeding or patients with renal insufficiency.
- **Risk factors for GI bleeding:** age >65, oral steroids, history of peptic ulcer disease or GI bleeding, anticoagulation.
- **Risk factors for renal failure:** age >65, serum creatinine >2, HTN, congestive heart failure, diuretics, ACE inhibitors.

- **Tramadol (Ultram)** (50 mg PO q6h) can be used in patients who do not respond to APAP and are not candidates for NSAID therapy. Side effects: nausea, constipation, and drowsiness. Avoid in patients with a low seizure threshold.

- **Opioids** may be considered in patients who do not respond to NSAIDS or tramadol or who cannot tolerate these medications. See Chap. 24, Miscellaneous Subjects, for additional discussion of pain management.

- **Capsaicin cream** applied topically qid is a useful adjunct to oral analgesic therapy.

- Pain medications should be taken around the clock until pain relief is achieved, then taper to a prn basis.

- **Intraarticular injections** with hyaluronic acid or steroids (e.g., triamcinolone, 40 mg) are useful for patients who have acute pain in a single joint or contraindications to oral medications or who have not responded to oral therapy.

- **Oral glucosamine/chondroitin sulfate,** 1500 mg PO qd, has been shown to be effective for OA in limited studies (no strong randomized clinical trials using these agents).

- **Surgery** (total knee or total hip replacement) is an option for severe OA that has not responded to medical management.

When to Refer

- Refer to a rheumatologist for patients who do not respond to therapy.
- Refer to an orthopedic surgeon for surgery. Indications for surgery: Radiographic evidence of joint damage and moderate to severe persistent pain or disability that does not respond to medical management.

What to Tell the Patient

- OA is a chronic disease for which symptomatic therapy is the initial treatment.
- An exercise program is an integral part of improving pain symptoms and mobility.

SUGGESTED READING

American College of Rheumatology Recommendations for the Medical Management of Osteoarthritis of the Hip and Knee. *Arthritis Rheum* 2000;43(9):1905–1915.

Anderson BC. *Office orthopedics for primary care*, 2nd ed. Philadelphia: WB Saunders, 1999.

Emmerson BT. The management of gout. *N Engl J Med* 1996;334(7):445–451.

Howell JM. *Emergency medicine*. Philadelphia: WB Saunders, 1998.

Singh D, et al. Plantar fasciitis. *BMJ* 1997;315:172–175.

Stiell IG, Greenberg GH, et al. A study to develop clinical decision rules for the use of radiography in acute ankle injuries. *Ann Emerg Med* 1992;21:384–390.

Wedmore, IS. Emergency department evaluation and treatment of ankle and foot injuries. *Emerg Med Clin North Am* 2000;18(1):85–113.

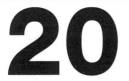# **Psychiatry**

I hate you, don't leave me . . .

GENERALIZED ANXIETY DISORDER
Epidemiology

- Depression and anxiety account for 13% of psychiatric cases seen in primary care.
- Up to 80% of patients with generalized anxiety disorder (GAD) also have depression. Approximately 55–60% of patients with GAD are women.

Key History

- **Symptoms:** excessive worry; cold, clammy hands; diaphoresis; dry mouth; choking sensation; palpitations; diarrhea; abdominal pain; tremor
- **Medical history:** Mood disorders (major depressive or dysthymic disorder), anxiety disorders (panic disorder, specific phobia, social phobia), substance-related disorders (alcohol or sedative, hypnotic or anxiolytic dependence or abuse)

Focused Physical Exam

- **Vital signs:** BP, pulse
- **General:** anxious appearing; fidgeting; cold, clammy hands

Evaluation

- Diagnosis is usually made by history and physical exam.
- Labs used to rule out medical conditions and drugs as causes of anxiety: TSH, urine drug screen.

Management

- **Nonpharmacologic:** relaxation techniques (massage, yoga), biofeedback, cognitive behavioral therapy
- **Pharmacologic:**
  - **Benzodiazepines:** Clonazepam (Klonopin), 0.5–2 mg PO bid–tid, for rapid control of anxiety until antidepressants start taking effect. Abuse potential. Comorbid substance abuse (alcohol, opiates) can be lethal.

- **Buspirone (BuSpar):** Start at 7.5 mg PO bid, can titrate to 15 mg PO tid.

- **SSRIs:** Paroxetine (Paxil), 20–40 mg PO qd or sertraline (Zoloft), 50–100 mg PO qd. May worsen anxiety initially but provide good long-term control of anxiety. No abuse potential. Side effects: sexual dysfunction, weight gain.

- **Venlafaxine (Effexor XR):** 37.5–225 mg PO qd. Monitor BP; can cause HTN or impair control of existing HTN. Sudden discontinuation or dose reduction causes a withdrawal syndrome.

- **Start low, go slow.** Rapid titration can lead to noncompliance because of side effects.

When to Refer

Consider referral to a psychiatrist when excessive anxiety and worry are possibly due to complex psychiatric diagnoses.

What to Tell the Patient

- GAD is a common diagnosis and is easily treatable.

- Two types of medication are usually prescribed. Benzodiazepines are used to control anxiety initially; antidepressants are prescribed for long-term control. Caution patients that benzodiazepines have abuse potential and are for *short-term* use only.

- Remission is defined as the improvement of ≥50% of symptoms for a 12-mo time period. Medication discontinuation with slow taper may be possible if a patient stays in remission for 12 mos.

DEPRESSION
Key History

- **Psychiatric symptoms present for ≥2 wks** with many of the following features:

  - Depressed mood

  - Feelings of worthlessness, helplessness, guilt, hopelessness

  - Anhedonia

  - Sleep disturbances (middle and terminal insomnia)

  - Decreased initiative, concentration, energy, motivation

  - Psychomotor retardation/agitation

  - Increased or decreased appetite

  - *Suicidality*: Assess for frequency, intensity, and lethality of thoughts

- Does the patient have a plan?
- Does the patient have access to materials that could be used for suicide (gun, medications)?
- Last suicide attempt, reasons for attempt, mechanism of attempt?
- What is preventing the patient from attempting suicide at present?

- **Medical history:** chronic disease (e.g., diabetes, coronary artery disease, HIV, malignancy), depression, other mental illness
- **Medications:** beta blockers, interferon, current and prior antidepressants
- **Family history:** depression, suicidality
- **Social history:** elevated stress (marital, financial, work-related), alcohol use, drug use, sexual/physical abuse, lack of support system

Focused Mental Status Exam

- **Appearance:** poor hygiene, disheveled
- **Mood:** description of how patient feels
- **Affect:** expression of mood
- **Speech:** rate, volume, frequency, tone
- **Thought processing:** logical and goal-directed conversation
- **Thought content:** "themes" underlying patient's perception of life
- **Perceptual disturbances:** auditory or visual hallucinations, dissociative or depersonalization episodes
- **Insight:** patient's understanding of illness
- **Judgment:** patient's decision-making capability, patient safety
- **Motivation:** patient's interest in treatment

Evaluation

***DSM-IV* criteria for major depressive disorder:** depression or anhedonia and ≥5 of the following symptoms present for ≥2 wks: **S**leep, **I**nterest (lack of), **G**uilt, **E**nergy, **C**oncentration, **A**ppetite, **P**sychomotor retardation, **S**uicide **(SIG E CAPS).**

- **Labs** to rule out medical causes of depression: CBC, electrolytes, LFTs, TSH, UA

- **Urine drug screen** if suspected substance abuse
- **ECG** before starting any medication to rule out QT prolongation
- Major depression cannot be diagnosed if depressed mood is because of
  - A direct effect of drug abuse
  - A side effect of medication or treatment
  - A toxin exposure
  - A direct physiologic effect of a general medical condition
  - Bereavement

Management

- *The most serious consequence of a major depressive episode is suicide. Any patient with suicidal ideation needs prompt evaluation by a psychiatrist!*
- **Medications:**
  - Start at a low dose; titrate to effect. May take several weeks to see improvement.
  - Almost all medications should be tapered slowly to avoid withdrawal symptoms.
  - **First-line therapy is with SSRIs:**
    - Paroxetine (Paxil), 10 mg PO qd; sertraline (Zoloft), 50 mg PO qd; citalopram (Celexa), 20 mg PO qd; fluoxetine (Prozac), 20 mg PO qd.
    - Side effects: insomnia, diarrhea, anorexia, anxiety, sexual dysfunction.
    - All SSRIs (except citalopram) have significant drug–drug interactions.
  - **Other medication classes:**
    - **Dopamine reuptake inhibitors:** bupropion SR (Wellbutrin SR), 150 mg PO qd. Side effects: seizures, arrhythmias, agitation, dry mouth, weight gain. No sexual side effects.
    - **Serotonin-norepinephrine reuptake inhibitors:** nefazodone (Serzone), 100 mg PO bid; trazodone (Desyrel), 150 mg PO qhs. Side effects: sedation, dizziness, dry mouth, nausea, vomiting.

- **Norepinephrine reuptake inhibitor:** venlafaxine XR (Effexor XR), 75 mg PO qd. Side effects: seizures, headache, somnolence, weight loss, anorexia, dizziness, dry mouth, sexual dysfunction.

- **Norepinephrine/selective serotonin receptor antagonist:** mirtazapine (Remeron), 15 mg PO qhs. Side effects: somnolence, dry mouth, weight gain, dizziness, agranulocytosis. Useful in combination therapy with SSRI, particularly if insomnia is an issue.

- **Tricyclic antidepressants:** not used frequently as monotherapy for depression because of side effects and risk of potential lethal overdose.

- Consider **referral for counseling** (individual, couples, marital) if appropriate.

When to Refer

- **Immediate referral to the ED is required for patients with suicidal or homicidal ideation.**

- Refer to a psychiatrist if:

  - Recurrent or severe depression.

  - Patient does not respond to one or two drugs from different classes, given in maximum doses for 6–8 wks.

  - Comorbid dual diagnosis (e.g., depression and alcoholism).

  - Depressive disorder due to toxin exposure, medical problems, or other medication is under consideration.

  - Person has psychotic features with depressed mood (delusions, hallucinations).

What to Tell the Patient

- Depressive disorders are frequent and appear at all ages, with a prevalence of 3% in the general population.

- Depression is a medical illness, not a character defect or weakness. Recovery is the rule, not the exception.

- Treatments are effective, and many options are available.

- Risk of recurrence on medication discontinuation is high (50% after one episode, 70% after two, 90% after three), so medications likely need to be taken on a long-term basis.

- Patients and their families should be alert for early signs and symptoms of recurrence and seek help early.

SUGGESTED READING

Delgado PL. Approaches to enhancement of patient adherence to antidepressant therapy. *J Clin Psychiatry* 2000;61(Suppl 2):6–9.

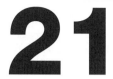

Pulmonary

Take a deep breath . . .

DYSPNEA

Dyspnea is a subjective experience of discomfort manifested as shortness of breath.

Differential Diagnosis

Cardiac

- Angina
- Cardiac asthma
- Cardiac tamponade
- Congestive heart failure (CHF)
- MI
- Valvular disease

Pulmonary

- Asthma
- Chronic bronchitis/COPD
- Infections
- Interstitial lung disease
- Pneumothorax
- Pulmonary edema
- Pulmonary embolism
- Pulmonary fibrosis

Other

- Anemia
- Ascites
- Neuromuscular diseases
- Panic attack/anxiety
- Pregnancy

Key History

- **General:** symptom onset, episodic vs constant, exacerbating/relieving factors, sick contacts, deep venous thrombosis risk factors

- **Cardiovascular:** chest pain/tightness

- **Pulmonary:** chest tightness, constriction, increased work of breathing, air hunger, rapid-shallow breaths, smothering/suffocation, labored breathing, hemoptysis, cough, pleuritic chest pain

- **GI:** GERD symptoms, hiatal hernia

- **Musculoskeletal:** associated muscle, bone pain

- **Medical history:** pulmonary pathology (e.g., asthma, emphysema, bronchitis, bronchiectasis), CHF, coronary artery disease, neurologic illness, deep venous thrombosis/pulmonary embolism, anemia

- **Social history:** smoking history, exercise capacity, assessment of activities of daily living, recent travel

- **Occupational exposures:** exposure to fumes (patients with occupational exposures typically have symptoms that correlate with the workweek and resolve over the weekends), chemicals, asbestos, beryllium, silicone

Focused Physical Exam

- **Vital signs:** temperature, BP, heart rate, respiratory rate, O_2 saturation

- **General:** fatigue, pallor, fever/chills, peripheral/central cyanosis, amount of respiratory distress

- **HEENT:** pale conjunctiva, elevated jugular venous pulse, lymphadenopathy

- **Cardiovascular:** rate, murmurs, gallops

- **Pulmonary:** crackles, wheezing, stridor, ventilatory effort, accessory muscle use

- **Abdominal:** ascites

- **Extremities:** peripheral edema, digital clubbing

- **Neurologic:** paralysis or deficit

Evaluation

- **Labs:** consider CBC, Chem 7, TSH, D-dimer (to evaluate for pulmonary embolus)

- **Pulse oximetry:** O_2 saturation reflects the percentage of oxyhemoglobin in the blood, but does not measure ventilation (i.e., CO_2).

- **Arterial blood gases:** pH, PaO_2, $PaCO_2$. Used to assess the nature and severity of the patient's dyspnea. Consider if suspect hypercarbia or hypoxemia.

- **Pulmonary function tests (PFTs):** consider to assess severity of pulmonary processes and evaluate the possibility of a pulmonary cause for dyspnea; interval evaluations to assess progression of disease. Not indicated in active acute processes, such as TB, asthmatic exacerbation, or active hemoptysis.

- **Chest x-ray:** consider to assess for cardiomegaly suggestive of CHF, pneumothorax, and interstitial lung diseases, such as fibrosis, emphysema, and TB.

- **Ventilation-perfusion scan:** consider to test for pulmonary emboli. A clear chest x-ray improves interpretability of the scan.

- **Chest CT:** consider to assess lung parenchyma, mediastinum, and upper abdomen. Spiral CT can evaluate for pulmonary emboli also.

- **Cardiopulmonary exercise:** consider to evaluate unexplained exertional dyspnea. Determines minute ventilation, expired oxygen and carbon dioxide, heart rate, BP, and respiratory rate.

- **Two-dimensional (2D) echocardiography:** consider to detect valvular abnormalities, the ejection fraction, the presence of intracardiac shunts, and indirect measurements of pulmonary artery pressures.

- **Cardiac stress testing (treadmill, nuclear, echo):** consider to evaluate for cardiac ischemia. See Chap. 22, Coronary Artery Disease.

Management

- Treat the underlying cause of the patient's dyspnea.

- Please refer to the appropriate sections of this chapter (e.g., Chronic Obstructive Pulmonary Disease; Asthma; Congestive Heart Failure; Coronary Artery Disease) for details on management.

ASTHMA
Differential Diagnosis

- **Pulmonary:** chemical pneumonitis, COPD, upper airway obstruction (tumor, tracheomalacia), Churg-Strauss syndrome, allergic bronchopulmonary aspergillosis, hypersensitivity pneumonitis

- **Other:** GERD, CHF, anxiety disorder/panic attacks, vocal cord dysfunction

Key History

- **History of present illness:** timing of symptoms, factors that exacerbate symptoms (exercise, allergies), response to bronchodilator therapy, nighttime symptoms, need for steroids, number of exacerbations

- **HEENT:** rhinorrhea

- **Pulmonary:** shortness of breath, cough (nighttime symptoms)
- **Medical history:** hospitalizations/intubations, previous treatment, environmental allergies (dust mites, trees, grass, flowers), other atopic disorders (eczema), chemical exposures, anxiety disorder, sinusitis, GERD
- **Medications:** beta blockers, NSAIDs, ASA (especially in association with nasal polyps), ACE inhibitors, inhaled pentamidine, compliance with medications, appropriate use of inhalers
- **Family history:** atopy, asthma, eczema
- **Social history:** sports activities, tobacco use, drug use, home environment (pets, dust, age of home, carpets, bedding), occupational exposures (chemicals, dust)

Focused Physical Exam

- **Vital signs:** temperature, BP, heart rate, respiratory rate
- **General:** accessory muscle use
- **HEENT:** nasal polyps, sinus pain, ocular injection, nasal discharge, boggy nasal turbinates
- **Cardiovascular:** tachycardia, jugular venous distention
- **Pulmonary:** dyspnea, tachypnea, wheezing, absence of wheezing in a very distressed patient (ominous sign), rales, decreased breath sounds, stridor, expiratory phase, decreased peak flows
- **Skin:** rash (eczema)

Evaluation

- Check **peak flows** to assess baseline dysfunction.
- **Baseline PFTs** with bronchodilators (need increase in FEV_1 >12% and 200 cc for diagnosis of asthma); consider adding methacholine challenge for patients who have symptoms consistent with asthma but who do not meet PFT criteria for diagnosis.
- **Chest x-ray**
- **Labs:** CBC with differential, especially looking for infection (not consistent with asthma) or eosinophilia (more consistent with asthma/allergies).
- **Skin test** for atopy (if indicated by history).

Management

- See **Table 21-1** for classification of asthma. Recommended treatment **(Table 21-2)** is based on classification; place patients in the category of their most severe symptom or feature.

TABLE 21-1.
ASTHMA CLASSIFICATION

Classification	Symptoms	Nighttime symptoms	Lung function
Mild inter-mittent	Symptoms <2×/wk. Asymptomatic and normal peak flows between exac-erbations. Exacerbations brief; inten-sity may vary.	<2×/mo	FEV_1 or PEF >80% predicted PEF variability <20%
Mild persis-tent	Symptoms >2×/wk but <1×/day. Exacerbations may affect activity.	>2×/mo	FEV_1 or PEF >80% predicted PEF variability 20–30%
Moderate persistent	Daily symptoms. Daily use of inhaled short-acting beta$_2$-agonist. Exacerbations affect activity. Exacerbations >2×/wk; may last days.	>1×/wk	FEV_1 or PEF 60–80% PEF variability >30%
Severe per-sistent	Continual symptoms. Limited physical activity. Frequent exacerbations.	Frequent	FEV_1 or PEF <60% of predicted PEF variability >30%
Status asth-maticus	Severe, continuous bron-chospasm	—	—

PEF, peak expiratory flow.
Based on *NAEPP Expert Panel Report: guidelines for the diagnosis and management of asthma*. NIH Publication 02-5075, 2002.

- **Lifestyle modifications:**

  - Have patient check peak flows daily in morning before taking medications; take best of three measurements to assess daily lung functions.

  - Avoid trigger factors.

  - For environmental allergies, cover mattresses and pillows with allergen-proof casings, or wash bedding in ≥130°F water 1×/wk. May also consider eliminating carpeting, using dust filters, and removing pets.

  - Encourage regular exercise, with use of inhalers prophylactically if needed.

TABLE 21-2.
ASTHMA MANAGEMENT

Classification	Long-term control	Quick relief
Mild intermittent	No daily medication needed	Inhaled beta$_2$-agonist prn for symptoms
	Lifestyle modifications	If using short-acting inhaler >2×/wk, may need long-term control therapy
Mild persistent	Low-dose inhaled corticosteroid or cromolyn	Inhaled beta$_2$-agonist prn for symptoms
	May also consider sustained-release theophylline or leukotriene antagonist	If having increasing symptoms or increasing use of short-acting inhaler, may need additional long-term control therapy
	Lifestyle modifications	
Moderate persistent	Inhaled corticosteroid (medium dose) **or**	Inhaled beta$_2$-agonist prn for symptoms
	Inhaled corticosteroid (low to medium dose) **plus** long-acting bronchodilator, especially for nighttime symptoms	If having increasing symptoms or increasing use of short-acting inhaler, may need additional long-term control therapy
	Lifestyle modifications	
Severe persistent	Inhaled corticosteroid (high dose) **plus**	Inhaled beta$_2$-agonist prn for symptoms
	Long-acting bronchodilator; may also need PO steroids	If having increasing symptoms or increasing use of short-acting inhaler, may need additional long-term control therapy
	Lifestyle modifications	
Status asthmaticus	Continuous nebulizer treatments	
	Epinephrine	
	O$_2$	
	Arrange transfer to ED	

Based on *NAEPP Expert Panel Report: guidelines for the diagnosis and management of asthma.* NIH Publication 02-5075, 2002.

- **Medications:**
- See Table 21-3 for proper metered-dose inhaler (MDI) technique.
  - **Inhaled corticosteroids:** See Table 21-4 for dosing information.
    - Rinse mouth after inhalations.

TABLE 21-3.
PROPER METERED-DOSE INHALER (MDI) TECHNIQUE

Shake inhaler.

Tilt head back slightly and exhale normally (forced exhalation to residual volume not necessary).

Hold mouthpiece 1–1.5 in. away from open mouth (if using a spacer, however, seal lips around the mouthpiece).

Activate MDI while simultaneously taking a slow, deep inhalation.

Hold breath at end of inspiration for 5–10 secs, then slowly exhale through mouth.

Wait 1 min between puffs.

If using steroid inhalers, rinse mouth after use to avoid thrush or dysphonia.

- Side effects: headache, throat irritations, hoarseness, oral candidiasis, cough.
- **Inhaled corticosteroid/beta$_2$ agonist combination**
  - **Fluticasone/salmeterol** (Advair Diskus 100/50, 250/50, 500/50), 1 inhalation bid.
  - Rinse mouth after inhalation.
  - Side effects: palpitations, upper respiratory tract infections, cough, pharyngitis, headache.

TABLE 21-4.
INHALED CORTICOSTEROID DOSAGES FOR ASTHMA

Drug	Low dose	Medium dose	High dose
Budesonide (Pulmicort), 200 µg/dose	200–400 µg, 1–2 inhalations/day	400–600 µg, 2–3 inhalations/day	>600 µg, >3 inhalations/day
Flunisolide (AeroBid), 250 µg/puff	500–1000 µg, 2–4 puffs/day	1000–2000 µg, 4–8 puffs/day	>2000 µg, >8 puffs/day
Fluticasone (Flovent)	88–264 µg	264–660 µg	>660 µg
MDI: 44, 110, 220 µg/puff	2–3 puffs/day	2–6 puffs/day	>3–6 puffs/day
DPI: 50, 100, 250 µg/dose	2–6 inhalations/day	3–6 inhalations/day	>6 inhalations/day
Triamcinolone (Vanceril), 100 µg/puff	400–1000 µg, 4–10 puffs/day	1000–2000 µg, 10–20 puffs/day	>2000 µg, >20 puffs/day

From *NAEPP Expert Panel Report: guidelines for the diagnosis and management of asthma*. NIH Publication 02-5075, 2002.

- **Beta$_2$ agonists**
  - **Albuterol MDI,** 2 puffs q4h prn (as rescue inhaler)
  - **Albuterol,** 2.5 mg nebulized tid–qid (consider this option for those who have difficulty with MDI technique)
  - **Salmeterol MDI,** 2 puffs bid (not for acute bronchospasm, but for longer-term control)
  - Side effects: palpitations, tremor, tachycardia, nervousness, dizziness, insomnia, cough, throat irritation

- **Leukotriene inhibitors:**
  - Adjunct to inhalers, consider adding if patient is difficult to control with inhalers alone. Useful for patients with ASA intolerance, nighttime symptoms, or exercise-induced asthma.
  - **Montelukast** (Singulair), 10 mg PO qd, or **zafirlukast** (Accolate), 20 mg PO bid
  - Side effects: headache, nausea, diarrhea, rhinitis, elevated LFTs, dyspepsia, abdominal pain, myalgias, angioedema, urticaria, rare eosinophilia

- **Oral corticosteroids:**
  - For acute exacerbation, start **prednisone,** 40–60 mg PO qd; taper over 5–7 days.
  - Side effects (primarily long term): osteoporosis, immunosuppression, adrenal insufficiency, steroid psychosis, peptic ulcer disease, headache, dizziness, mood swings, anxiety, cushingoid features, hyperglycemia, menstrual irregularities, acne, skin atrophy.

- **Theophylline:**
  - Not routinely used as first-line therapy. Consider if patient is poorly responsive to other medications.
  - Dose is 100–300 mg PO bid. Must monitor levels.
  - Side effects: seizures, arrhythmias, nausea, headache, vomiting, insomnia, nervousness, tremor, tachycardia, palpitations.

- **Management of exercise-induced asthma:**
  - Treat like mild, intermittent asthma.
  - **Albuterol,** 3 puffs 20 mins before exercise, is generally sufficient to prevent symptoms.

Difficult Management Situations

- Bronchospasm can be exacerbated by many conditions, including seasonal allergies and GERD. Consider adding an antihistamine for allergic symptoms or an H$_2$-blocker for GERD symptoms if indicated.

- Other conditions that can mimic refractory asthma: CHF, tumors (endotracheal and endobronchial), tracheomalacia, allergic bronchopulmonary aspergillosis (particularly if symptoms were previously well controlled), vocal cord dysfunction, Churg-Strauss syndrome.

When to Refer

Refer to a pulmonologist for asthma that does not respond to therapy or patient experiencing frequent exacerbations despite treatment.

What to Tell the Patient

- Have a plan of action in place in case of exacerbations, including an extra dose of prednisone (20 mg) on hand.

  - **If peak flows ≥80% of maximum,** continue daily regimen as prescribed.

  - **If peak flows = 50–79% of maximum,** take 4 extra puffs of short-acting inhaler q1–2h prn and contact physician to be seen within 1–2 days.

  - **If peak flows <50% of maximum,** take 4 extra puffs of short-acting inhaler **AND** prednisone dose, go to ED immediately.

  - **If patient begins to have symptoms of severe dyspnea, use of neck and abdominal muscles to breathe, blue fingers/lips, the patient should go to the nearest ED immediately.**

- Consider referral to asthma nurse educator (if available in your clinic).

- Emphasize the importance of daily therapy to those who need it.

CHRONIC OBSTRUCTIVE PULMONARY DISEASE
Definition

- COPD is a **spectrum** of pulmonary disorders characterized by airway obstruction (impaired expiratory airflow) on spirometry.

- **Major subsets:**

  - **Chronic bronchitis:** cough and phlegm production for ≥3 mos/yr for 2 consecutive yrs

  - **Emphysema:** anatomic abnormality of lung with permanent enlargement of air spaces and destruction of walls, without obvious fibrosis

- Most patients exhibit features of **both** chronic bronchitis and emphysema.

Key History

- **General:** older (usually >50), fatigue, weight loss, decreased appetite, sleep disturbances

- **Pulmonary:** progressive dyspnea, decreased exercise tolerance, cough (onset before dyspnea, productive of whitish-gray sputum, worse in morning), wheezing (bronchospastic component), hemoptysis (underlying infection, malignancy)

- **Psychiatric:** depression, poor concentration, memory impairment

- **Family history:** alpha$_1$-antitrypsin deficiency

- **Social history:** smoking or former smoking adult (the most important factor in development of COPD), occupational exposures, missed work due to pulmonary symptoms

Focused Physical Exam

Vital Signs

- Chronic bronchitis ("blue bloaters"): normal respiratory rate

- Emphysema ("pink puffers"): tachypneic

General

- Chronic bronchitis ("blue bloaters"): normal or obese habitus, comfortable appearing

- Emphysema ("pink puffers"): cachectic/weight loss, uncomfortable appearing

HEENT

Chronic bronchitis ("blue bloaters"): nasal polyps, evidence of allergic rhinitis ("asthmatic bronchitis")

Pulmonary

- Chronic bronchitis ("blue bloaters"): resonant on percussion, wheezes, coarse rhonchi (may change location with cough)

- Emphysema ("pink puffers"): hyperresonant on percussion, increased breath sounds, accessory muscle use

Cardiovascular

- Chronic bronchitis ("blue bloaters"): cor pulmonale (distended neck veins, right ventricular heave, right ventricular gallop)

Extremities

- Chronic bronchitis ("blue bloaters"): cyanotic (blue), peripheral edema

- Emphysema ("pink puffers"): pink (until advanced)

Evaluation

- **PFTs:** For diagnosis and classification of COPD, see **Table 21-5.**

TABLE 21-5.
COPD CLASSIFICATION

Category	FEV$_1$ (%)
Mild COPD	80–65
Moderate COPD	65–50
Severe COPD	<50

- **FEV$_1$/FVC** (ratio of 1-sec forced expiratory volume to vital capacity): below the predicted value
- **FEV$_1$** (forced expiratory volume in 1 sec): most predictive of prognosis, used to categorize disease severity
- **Decrease in FEF$_{25-75}$** not diagnostic but indicates obstruction of the small airways
- **Decrease in D$_{LCO}$:** more prominent in emphysema vs chronic bronchitis or asthmatic bronchitis
- Increase in **TLC and RV:** more prominent in emphysema; indicative of "air trapping"
- **Bronchodilator response:**
  - Positive if >12% and >200 cc increase in FEV$_1$ or FVC
  - Normalization of FEV$_1$/FVC suggests asthma rather than COPD
- **Exercise testing** usually not indicated
- **Chest x-ray:**
  - **Emphysema predominant:** hyperexpanded lung fields, flattened diaphragms, increased anterior-posterior diameter, apical bullae with increased vascular markings
  - **Bronchitis-predominant:** increased interstitial markings ("dirty lungs")
  - Bullae of the lower lobes in younger patient suggests alpha$_1$-antitrypsin deficiency
- **ABG:**
  - Usually normal early in disease
  - Hypoxemia (decrease Pa$_{O_2}$) and hypercapnia (increase Pa$_{CO_2}$) during exacerbations or advanced disease (especially bronchitis predominant)
- **CBC with differential:** for polycythemia, eosinophilia (asthmatic bronchitis)

- **ECG:** for right atrial enlargement or right ventricular hypertrophy (cor pulmonale), sinus tachycardia, multifocal atrial tachycardia
- **Alpha$_1$-antitrypsin levels:** for suspected deficiency
- **Skin allergy tests** and **serum IgE:** for suspected asthmatic bronchitis

Management

- **Smoking cessation is the most important modification for patients.** (See Chap. 7, Health Maintenance and Disease Prevention)
- **Anticholinergics:**
  - **Ipratropium MDI**
    - First-line therapy (superior to beta$_2$ adrenergic agonists in bronchodilation)
    - Ipratropium, 2 puffs (18 µg/puff) qid; may increase to 3–6 puffs qid
  - **Ipratropium nebulizer:** 0.5 mg/2.5 mL NS neb q6–8h
- **Beta$_2$ agonists:**
  - Considered second-line therapy
  - **Albuterol MDI:** 1–2 puffs q4–6h; maximum, 2–6 puffs 4–6×/day
  - **Albuterol nebulizer:** 2.5 mg/5 mL neb q4–6h
    - Useful in conjunction with ipratropium (or replaces ipratropium in nonresponders)
    - Use during acute exacerbations
- **Combivent:**
  - Combines ipratropium and albuterol in a single MDI
  - Traditional dose: 2 puffs (120 µg albuterol/21 µg ipratropium) qid; maximum, 2–6 puffs 4–6×/day
  - More effective in improving FEV$_1$ than either agent alone (but not in subjective symptomatic improvement)
- **Home O$_2$ therapy** (indications for use based on Medicare requirements):
  - **Indications for continuous home O$_2$ therapy:**
    - Resting state, room air PaO$_2$ ≤55 mm Hg or SaO$_2$ ≤88%
    - Resting state, room air PaO$_2$ of 56–59 mm Hg or SaO$_2$ ≤89%, **in cases in which the** patient has polycythemia (Hct ≥52%), dependent edema (CHF), or ECG evidence of cor pulmonale (P pulmonale)

- **Indications for home O$_2$ for nocturnal therapy:**
  - During sleep, PaO$_2$ $\leq$55 mm Hg or SaO$_2$ $\leq$88%
  - Decrease PaO$_2$ >10 mm Hg or decrease SaO$_2$ >5% associated with hypoxemic symptoms (altered mental status, nocturnal restlessness/insomnia)
- **Indications for home O$_2$ during exercise:** PaO$_2$ $\leq$55 mm Hg or SaO$_2$ $\leq$88%, and evidence that O$_2$ improves hypoxemia.
- **Home O$_2$ is the only therapy shown to improve morbidity/mortality in COPD.**
- **Theophylline**
  - Considered a third-line agent. Consider use in suboptimal responders to ipratropium and beta$_2$ agonist MDIs.
  - Usual dose: Start 300–400 mg PO qd; titrate up to 600–900 mg PO qd if tolerated.
  - Monitor levels initially in 1–2 wks, then twice annually (goal, 8–12 µg/mL; >20 µg/mL toxic).
  - Clearance decreases with antibiotics (fluoroquinolones, clarithromycin), cimetidine, calcium channel blockers, liver disease, cor pulmonale, and pregnancy.
  - Side effects: nausea, diarrhea, tremor, anxiety, insomnia, seizures, arrhythmias.
- **Inhaled corticosteroids:** role in treatment is unclear (may be beneficial for patients with asthmatic bronchitis).
- **Systemic corticosteroids:**
  - Beginning dose: **prednisone,** 0.5–1 mg/kg PO qd.
  - Objectively benefit only 10% of clinically stable outpatients with COPD.
  - Obtain PFTs before initiation; repeat after 2 wks of treatment (assess for objective improvement in FEV$_1$; discontinue if no improvement).
- **Antibiotics:**
  - Treatment for acute infectious exacerbations of COPD, with concurrent change in sputum (appearance/quantity).
  - Common bugs: *Haemophilus influenzae, Streptococcus pneumoniae, Moraxella catarrhalis.*
  - Common antimicrobials: amoxicillin (Amoxil), amoxicillin/clavulanate (Augmentin), tetracycline, macrolides, TMP-SMX (Bactrim).
  - Viruses will still be very common respiratory offenders (as seen in patients without COPD).

- **Vaccines:**
  - **Influenza vaccination:** annually
  - **Pneumococcal vaccination:** administer once (regardless of age with chronic pulmonary condition); revaccinate once in 5 yrs if initial vaccination administered at <65 yrs.
- **Lung reduction surgery:** may be an option for selected patients

What to Tell the Patient

- **Smoking cessation** (at any age) will slow the annual decrement in lung function to that of a nonsmoker.
- **Preventive measures:**
  - Occupational or environmental air pollutants may trigger COPD exacerbations, especially if the patient has asthmatic bronchitis. Common irritants: aerosol deodorants, hairsprays, spray paints, and insecticides.
- **Technique for clearing airway secretions:** slow, deep breaths with 5- to 10-sec breath holding to increase intrathoracic pressure, then coughing on exhalation.
- **Comprehensive pulmonary rehabilitation** may optimize functional ability.
- **Air travel:** refer patients with a PaO_2 <70 on room air to evaluate need for and amount of O_2 supplementation during air travel.
- Instruct on proper MDI technique (Table 21-3).

COMMUNITY-ACQUIRED PNEUMONIA
Epidemiology

Common pathogens	Prevalence (%)
Streptococcus pneumoniae	30–75
Mycoplasma pneumoniae	5–35
Haemophilus influenzae	6–12
Staphylococcus aureus	3–10
Gram-negative organisms	3–10
Moraxella catarrhalis	0.5–1
Viruses	2–10

See also the Official Statement of the American Thoracic Society: Guidelines for the management of adults with community-acquired pneumonia. *Am J Resp Crit Care Med* 2001;163:1730–1754.

Key History

- **General:** fever, chills, sweats.

- **Pulmonary:** dyspnea, pleuritic chest pain, cough (dry or productive [sputum description], onset [acute or gradual]).

- Table 21-6 lists historical clues and associated organisms.

Specific Pathogen Risk Factors

- **Penicillin-resistant and drug-resistant pneumococci:** age >65, beta-lactam therapy (last 3 mos), alcoholism, corticosteroid use

TABLE 21-6.
COMMUNITY-ACQUIRED PNEUMONIA: HISTORICAL CLUES AND ASSOCIATED ORGANISMS

History	Likely organisms
Medical history:	
Healthy and young	*Mycoplasma, Streptococcus pneumoniae*
COPD/smoking	*S. pneumoniae, Haemophilus influenzae, M. catarrhalis, Legionella*
Diabetes	*Staphylococcus aureus, S. pneumoniae*
Sickle cell, asplenism	*S. pneumoniae, H. influenzae, S. aureus*
Postinfluenzal status	*S. aureus, S. pneumoniae*
Neutropenia	*S. aureus, S. pneumoniae*, gram (–) bacteria
HIV infection (late)	PCP, *Cryptococcus, Histoplasma capsulatum*
Seizures, decreased mental status	Oral organisms (aspiration)
Social history:	
Alcoholism	*S. pneumoniae, Klebsiella, S. aureus*
IV drug abuse	*S. aureus*
Homeless or incarcerated	Increased risk for TB
Environmental contacts	Birds (*C. psittaci*), livestock (*C. burnetii*), or rabbits (*Francisella tularensis*), bats (*H. capsulatum*)
Travel history	Southwestern U.S. (*Coccidioides*), Midwest (*Histoplasma*)
Nursing home resident	*S. pneumoniae,* gram (–) bacteria

PCP, *Pneumocystis carinii* pneumonia.

(>10 mg/day), children in day care, multiple comorbidities, immuno-suppressive illness

- **Enteric gram-negatives:** nursing home residence, cardiopulmonary disease, multiple comorbidities, recent antibiotic course

- ***Pseudomonas aeruginosa:*** structural lung disease (bronchiectasis), corticosteroids, broad-spectrum antibiotics (>7 days in the past mo), malnutrition

Focused Physical Exam

- **Vital signs:** fever/hypothermia, tachypnea/tachycardia.

- **HEENT:** periodontal disease (anaerobic organism).

- **Pulmonary:** crackles (also heard in bronchitis), consolidation (dullness to percussion, egophony, increased tactile fremitus), pleural effusions (dullness to percussion, decreased breath sounds, decreased tactile fremitus).

- **Neurologic:** mental status.

- **Skin:** erythema multiforme (*Mycoplasma pneumonia*), erythema nodosum (*Mycobacterium tuberculosis*, *Chlamydia* species, *Histoplasma capsulatum*, *Coccidioides immitis*).

- Exam may be unremarkable.

- Normal vital signs decrease probability of pneumonia in outpatients to <1%.

  - Pulse–temperature disparity (normal pulse despite high fever) may suggest *Mycoplasma, Legionella, Chlamydia,* or viral etiology.

Evaluation

- **A baseline chest x-ray** is recommended to

  - substantiate pneumonia diagnosis

  - detect associated lung diseases

  - provide a baseline to assess response

  - assess a pattern to possibly predict pathogen

  - evaluate for complications (pleural effusions, multilobar disease)

- **Sputum culture/Gram stain** (optional):

  - Deep cough specimen, obtain before antibiotics

  - Transport **immediately** to lab to optimize yield

- **Labs:** CBC, serum electrolytes, hepatic enzymes, renal function

TABLE 21-7.
EMPIRIC ANTIBIOTIC THERAPY IN OUTPATIENTS[a]

Patient subset	First line	Alternates
No cardiopulmonary disease (CHF, COPD), no modifying factors[b]	**Advanced-generation macrolide:** Azithromycin, 500 mg PO ×1 day, then 250 mg PO qd ×4 days or Clarithromycin, 500 mg PO bid, or XL, 1000 mg PO qd	Doxycycline, 100 mg PO bid
Cardiopulmonary disease and/or modifying factors[a]	**Option 1: Beta-lactam (see below) + macrolide (see above):** Cefpodoxime, 200 mg PO q12h or Cefuroxime, 500 mg PO q12h or Amoxicillin/clavulanate, 875 mg PO bid **Option 2: Respiratory fluoroquinolone:** Levofloxacin, 500 mg PO qd Gatifloxacin, 400 mg PO qd Moxifloxacin, 400 mg PO qd	Beta-lactam **and** doxycycline

[a]See also the Official Statement of the American Thoracic Society: Guidelines for the management of adults with community-acquired pneumonia. *Am J Resp Crit Care Med* 2001;163:1730–1754.
[b]Modifying factors: suspected *Streptococcus pneumoniae*, *Mycoplasma*, *Chlamydia*, *Legionella*, or *Haemophilus influenzae*.

Management

- Approximately 75% of pneumonia patients may be adequately managed as outpatients.

- **Patients who may need hospitalization:** age >65, coexisting chronic illness, abnormal vital signs

- Empiric antibiotic therapy in outpatients: see Table 21-7.

- **How long to treat:**

  - *S. pneumoniae* **pneumonia,** other typical bacterial organisms: 7–10 days

  - **Atypical organisms** (*Chlamydia, Mycoplasma, Legionella*): 10–14 days; **azithromycin is the exception:** 5 days (half-life is 11–14 hrs)

- **Supportive measures:**

  - Rest

- Adequate hydration (correct for fever-induced fluid loss)
- Analgesia

Difficult Management Situations
Considerations in the Nonresponding Patient

- May take 4–6 wks for infiltrates to clear on chest x-ray.
- Consider other diagnoses, including CHF, pulmonary embolism, malignancy, and sarcoid vasculitis.
- Possible drug issues: improper coverage, dosage error, and patient compliance.
- Consider complicated infections: obstruction, foreign body, empyema, immunosuppressed host.
- Pathogen issues: drug resistance, other atypical agents (mycobacteria, nocardia, fungi, viruses).

Further Evaluation of the Nonresponding Patient

- Consider additional tests, such as serologic tests for *Legionella*, *Mycoplasma*, viruses, endemic fungi, and urinary test for *Legionella* antigen.
- Consider nuclear scanning or chest CT for possible collections of pleural fluid, lung nodules, cavitation within a lung infiltrate, and chronic pulmonary embolism.
- All **parapneumonic effusions** warrant evaluation with thoracentesis.

What to Tell the Patient

- It is important to finish the prescribed course of antibiotics.
- Fever typically persists for 2–4 days.
- Notify physician if symptoms not improved after 3 days.
- Recommend appropriate vaccines (pneumococcal/flu).
- May continue to have nonspecific symptoms (cough, fatigue) for up to 1–2 mos after pneumonia.

COUGH
Differential Diagnosis

- **Acute (<3-wk duration):** upper respiratory infection (viral, postinfectious cough), COPD/asthma exacerbation, acute sinusitis (viral, bacterial), pneumonia, CHF exacerbation, aspiration, foreign body
- **Chronic (>3-wk duration):** postnasal drip (allergic rhinitis, vasomotor rhinitis, chronic sinusitis), GERD, chronic bronchitis, irritant exposure (smoking, chemicals, dry air), medications (e.g., ACE inhibitor),

CHF, TB, bronchiectasis, eosinophilic bronchitis, malignancy, rare causes (sarcoidosis, carcinomatosis, chronic aspiration, "nervous" or "habit" cough)

- **Cough with clear chest x-ray:** asthma, GERD, CHF, postnasal drip

Key History

- **General:** fever, weight loss, chills, night sweats (infection, malignancy)

- **HEENT:** rhinorrhea, sneezing, postnasal drip, nasal congestion, sore throat, hoarseness (URI, GERD), headache (sinusitis), maxillary toothache (bacterial sinusitis), purulent nasal secretion (bacterial sinusitis), sour brash/bitter taste in mouth (GERD)

- **Cardiovascular:** orthopnea, paroxysmal nocturnal dyspnea (CHF)

- **Pulmonary:**

  - Dyspnea (CHF, interstitial lung disease, malignancy, asthma/COPD)

  - Cough characteristics: duration, quality (barking, brassy), purulence (chronic infection, sinusitis, TB, bronchiectasis), blood (malignancy, TB, bronchiectasis)

  - Relation to food (alcohol, caffeine, GERD)

  - Positional (GERD, CHF)

- **GI:** heartburn (GERD)

- **Medications:** ACE inhibitors, H_2-blocker or proton pump inhibitor (GERD)

- **Family history:** asthma, atopy, allergies

- **Social history:** tobacco use, work/home environment (dust, chemicals, pets), TB/sick exposures

Focused Physical Exam

- **Vital signs:** fever (infection), weight loss (TB, malignancy)

- **HEENT:** sinus transillumination (acute bacterial sinusitis), cobblestoning of nasal mucosa (allergic rhinitis), nasal polyps (asthma), sinus tenderness/facial pain (sinusitis)

- **Pulmonary:** barrel chest (COPD), clear (URI, allergic rhinitis), wheezes (COPD, asthma), rhonchi (bronchitis), consolidation (pneumonia)

- **Cardiovascular:** S_3 gallop, edema, jugular venous distention, pulsatile/enlarged liver (CHF)

- **Skin:** eczema (asthma)

Evaluation

Suspected diagnosis	Suggested test(s)
Bacterial infection	CXR (rule out pneumonia)
Allergic rhinitis	Skin testing
Aspiration	CXR, swallow study
Asthma/COPD	CXR, pulmonary function tests
CHF	CXR, 2D echocardiogram
Chronic bronchitis	CXR
GERD	Empiric trial of PPI, 24-hr pH monitor
Interstitial lung disease	CXR, chest CT, biopsy
Malignancy	CXR, chest CT, biopsy
Sinusitis (chronic)	Limited sinus CT
TB	CXR, PPD

Management

- **Stopping smoking is the most important lifestyle modification for patients.**
- **Acute infection (viral syndrome):**
  - Empiric therapy with cough suppressant: dextromethorphan, 10–20 mg PO q4h, or sustained-release liquid, 60 mg PO q12h; can also try Robitussin AC (with codeine) or Tussionex (with hydrocodone).
  - Cough may last for several weeks after acute infection resolves (postinfectious cough).
- **Asthma or COPD exacerbation:**
  - Consider adding or increasing inhaled steroids or long-acting beta$_2$ agonist.
  - For COPD, consider ipratropium/albuterol (Combivent) inhaler, 4 puffs qid.
  - Consider prednisone taper (prednisone, 60 mg PO qd ×3 days, then 40 mg PO qd ×3 days, then 20 mg PO qd ×3 days, then 15 mg PO qd ×2days, then 10 mg PO qd ×2 days, then 5 mg PO qd ×2 days).
  - Antibiotics may be beneficial in COPD exacerbations; use clinical judgment.

- Consider admission to hospital for severe exacerbations of asthma or COPD.

- **Allergic rhinitis:**

  - See also Chap. 11, Ear, Nose, and Throat Diseases.

  - Antihistamines: loratadine (Claritin), 10 mg PO qd; cetirizine (Zyrtec), 10 mg PO qd; or fexofenadine (Allegra), 180 mg PO qd.

  - Nasal preparations can also be helpful: budesonide (Rhinocort) or fluticasone (Flonase), 2 sprays/nostril qd or nonsteroid spray azelastine (Astelin), 2 sprays/nostril bid.

- **CHF:** See Chap. 8, Congestive Heart Failure.

- **Chronic bronchitis:**

  - Eliminate irritant; cough will improve/resolve in 94–100% of patients with cessation of smoking.

  - Ipratropium (Atrovent), 2 puffs qid.

- **GERD:** See Chap. 13, Gastroenterology.

- **Medications:**

  - Discontinue ACE inhibitor. Cough should improve within 4 wks; otherwise, drug is not likely the cause of the cough. If it is, switch to angiotensin-receptor blocker.

- **Postnasal drip:**

  - See Chap. 11, Ear, Nose, and Throat Diseases.

- Sinusitis

  - See also Chap. 11, Ear, Nose, and Throat Diseases.

  - Viral: decongestants such as pseudoephedrine (Sudafed), 120 mg PO bid, or combination antihistamine/decongestants (Claritin-D, Allegra-D, Zyrtec-D).

  - Bacterial: antibiotic course (consider amoxicillin, Augmentin, fluoroquinolones) ×10–14 days, or 21-day course for chronic sinusitis.

  - Nasal sprays are also helpful: oxymetolazone (Afrin), 2 sprays/nostril bid; **use no more than 3 days total to avoid rebound congestion.** Nasal steroids (Flonase, 2 sprays/nostril qd) may also be beneficial.

- **Other cough suppression:**

  - Codeine, 8–15 mg PO q3–4h.

- Benzonatate (Tessalon Perles), 100 mg PO tid; caution patients about not chewing tablets and about side effects, including dizziness, nausea, chest numbness, and burning of eyes.

- Guaifenesin, 600–1200 mg PO bid, alone (mucolytic, not cough suppressant), or AC (codeine), DM (dextromethorphan), CF (DM/phenylpropanolamine), PE (phenylephrine), PAC (codeine/phenylephrine).

When to Refer

Consider referral to otolaryngologist (sinusitis, postnasal drip), pulmonologist (asthma, COPD, malignancy, TB, interstitial lung disease), allergist (allergic rhinitis, sinusitis), or cardiologist (CHF), depending on etiology.

What to Tell the Patient

- Chronic cough has many causes; it may take some investigation to determine cause of a cough.

- Return to the office if cough does not improve with treatment.

SLEEP-RELATED BREATHING DISORDERS
Definitions

- **Apnea:** cessation of airflow at nose/mouth for ≥10 secs.

- **Hypopnea:** decrement in airflow of ≥40–50% or a 4% fall in O_2 saturation or electroencephalographic arousal.

- **RDI** (respiratory disturbance index) = the number of *apneic + hypopneic* episodes/hr.

  - RDI is typically determined by a full night of polysomnography.

  - The RDI of 5–15 is required to make the diagnosis of a sleep-related breathing disorder.

  - Pathology increases with rising RDI.

- **Classes of apnea:**

  - **Central:** both airflow and respiratory effort are absent.

  - **Obstructive:** continued respiratory effort without airflow.

  - **Mixed:** central apnea that becomes obstructive in the same episode.

Differential Diagnosis

- **Primary sleep disorders:** obstructive sleep apnea, upper-airway resistance syndrome, obesity hypoventilation syndrome, Pickwickian syndrome, idiopathic central sleep apnea, primary alveolar hypoventilation (Ondine's curse)

- **Other causes of sleep disorders:** chest wall deformities (kyphoscoliosis), neuromuscular disorders, central alveolar hypoventilation (e.g., Shy-Drager syndrome, meningitis or encephalitis, MS and primary brain stem lesions), Cheyne-Stokes respiration

Risk Factors for Sleep Disorders

- Gender (male:female is 2:1)
- Obesity (>120% ideal body weight)
- Neck size (circumference at cricothyroid membrane >17" male and >15" female)
- Genetic diseases associated with craniofacial abnormalities: Down syndrome, achondroplasia
- Use of CNS depressants
- Nose abnormalities (septal abnormalities, nasal polyposis)
- Nasopharyngeal disease: carcinoma, adenoidal hypertrophy, pharyngeal flap, papillomatosis
- Mouth and oropharynx abnormalities: hypertrophic tonsils, lymphoma of tonsils, macroglossia, acromegaly, micrognathia, retrognathia, neck lipoma
- Neuromuscular disorders: cerebral palsy, myotonic dystrophy, muscular dystrophy, myasthenia gravis, MS, hypothyroidism, Chiari malformation, Shy-Drager syndrome
- Dysautonomia: olivopontocerebellar degeneration
- Spinal cord injuries: Bulbar stroke
- Neurologic injuries (cortical injury)

Key History

- **General:** hypersomnolence, daytime sleepiness, fatigue, obesity
- **Sleep history:** loud snoring (all patients with obstructive sleep apnea, often reported by bed partner); witnessed episodes of apnea, choking, or gasping during sleep; unrefreshing sleep; abnormal motor activity during sleep; insomnia
- **Cardiovascular:** nocturnal cardiac arrhythmias
- **Genitourinary:** nocturia, sexual impotence

TABLE 21-8.
EPWORTH SLEEPINESS SCALE

Scale: 0 = would never doze; 1 = slight chance of dozing; 2 = moderate chance of dozing; 3 = high chance of dozing

Based on your usual life, how likely are you to doze off or fall asleep in the following situations?

___ Sitting and reading

___ Watching TV

___ Sitting inactive in a public place (e.g., theater or meeting)

___ As a passenger in a car for an hour without a break

___ Sitting and talking to someone

___ Sitting quietly after lunch without alcohol

___ In a car, while stopped for a few minutes in traffic

Total score: _____

Score: <10 = normal, >10 = abnormal

Adapted from Johns MW. A new method for measuring daytime sleepiness. *Sleep* 1991;14:540–545.

- **Neurologic:** depression, irritability, impaired intellectual performance, morning headache
- **Medical history:** see risk factors on page 263; also HTN, coronary heart disease, cor pulmonale, pulmonary HTN, CHF
- **Medications:** CNS depressants
- **Social history:** automobile or industrial accident

Focused Physical Exam

- **Vital signs:** increased BP, increased weight.
- **General:** obesity.
- **HEENT:** narrow high-arching palate (may be present in 70% of patients); enlarged uvula, enlarged tonsils, pharyngeal crowding, drape-like soft palate.
- **Neck:** thick neck (>16 in.), jugular venous distention.
- **Cardiovascular:** rate, rhythm, right ventricular heave (cor pulmonale).
- **Pulmonary:** crackles.
- **Abdominal:** truncal obesity (may be present in 70% of patients).

• *Physical exam may be entirely normal.*

Evaluation

• **Epworth Sleepiness Scale** (Table 21-8): screen for daytime somnolence.

• **Labs:** CBC (polycythemia), ABG (hypercapnia, hypoxemia), pulse oximetry (hypoxia), TSH.

• **Full-night attended polysomnography:** Standard for diagnosis of sleep-related breathing disorders. RDI of >15 events/hr in the presence of both daytime and nighttime symptoms is also an accepted criteria for diagnosing obstructive sleep apnea.

Diagnosis of Obstructive Sleep Apnea*

• The patient has a complaint of excessive sleepiness or insomnia.

• Frequent episodes of obstructed breathing during sleep.

• The patient may be unaware of clinical features that are observed by others.

• Associated features include:

  • loud snoring

  • morning headaches

  • dry mouth on awakening

  • chest retraction during sleep in young children

• Polysomnographic monitoring demonstrates:

  • >5 obstructive apneas/hr that are >10 secs in duration and ≥1 of the following: frequent arousals from sleep associated with the apneas, bradytachycardia, or arterial oxygen desaturation in association with the apneic episodes

  • With or without a multisleep latency test that demonstrates a mean sleep latency of <10 mins

• Can be associated with other medical disorders (thyroid disease).

• Other sleep disorders can be present (periodic limb movement disorder or narcolepsy).

---

*From Diagnostic Classification Steering Committee. *The international classification of sleep disorders: diagnostic and coding manual*, 2nd ed. Lawrence, KS: Allen Press, 1997.

Management

- Therapy may be as basic as **modifying sleeping position** to lateral decubitus or wearing oral appliances at night.

- **Lifestyle modifications:** weight loss (decrease size of airway), avoidance of alcohol and sedatives (decreased pharyngeal-dilator muscle tone).

- **Screen for pathologic conditions** that may promote sleep apnea; may identify treatable conditions.

- **Positive pressure ventilation** at night (continuous positive airway pressure or bilevel positive airway pressure) may be indicated. Patients need a formal sleep study before positive pressure ventilation can be initiated.

- **Surgical treatment** may be helpful for certain patients.

When to Refer

- Refer to a sleep specialist any patient in whom you suspect a sleep disorder.

- **The patient should not drive until the sleep disorder is treated or excluded.**

What to Tell the Patient

- Consequences of sleep disorders are potentially serious and include increased BP and increased risk of MI, arrhythmias, cor pulmonale, hypersomnolence leading to cognitive decline, car accidents.

SUGGESTED READING

American Thoracic Society. Standards for the diagnosis and care of patients with chronic obstructive pulmonary disease. *Am J Respir Crit Care Med* 1995;152:S77–S121.

Barnes PJ. Chronic obstructive pulmonary disease. *N Engl J Med* 2000; 343:269–280.

Barnes PJ. New therapies for chronic obstructive pulmonary disease. *Thorax* 1998;53:137–147.

Bartlett JG. Practice guidelines for the management of community-acquired pneumonia in adults. Infectious Diseases Society of America. *Clin Infect Dis* 2000;31(2):347–382.

Marrie TJ, et al. A controlled trial of a critical pathway for treatment of community-acquired pneumonia. *JAMA* 2000;283(2):749–755.

National Asthma Education and Prevention Program: *Expert panel report 2: guidelines for diagnosis and management of asthma.* Bethesda,

MD, May 1997. National Institutes of Health. NIH Publication No. 97-4051A.

Official Statement of the American Thoracic Society: Guidelines for the management of adults with community-acquired pneumonia. *Am J Resp Crit Care Med* 2001;163:1730–1754.

Piccirillo J, Duntley S, Schotland H. Obstructive sleep apnea. *JAMA* 2000; 284:1492–1494.

Schwab RJ, Goldberg AN, Pack AI. Sleep apnea syndromes. In: Fishman A, Elias JA, et al., eds. *Fishman's pulmonary diseases and disorders*. New York: McGraw-Hill, 1998;1617–1637.

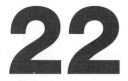

Renal Diseases

Spill the beans . . .

ACUTE RENAL FAILURE

Definition

An acute decline in glomerular filtration rate (GFR) from baseline (generally manifested as an increase in serum creatinine).

Etiology

Causes of acute renal failure (ARF) can be divided into three broad categories.

Prerenal Azotemia

- Decrease in effective perfusion of the renal vasculature.
- Caused by decreased cardiac output, hypovolemia, decreased effective circulating volume (e.g., cirrhosis).
- Kidneys sense a decreased volume status and avidly reabsorb Na^+ and water.
- Fractional excretion of Na^+ (FE_{Na}) is characteristically <1% (particularly if oliguric).

Intrinsic Azotemia

- Caused by renal parenchymal disease.
- Etiologies:
  - Vascular (atheroembolic disease, vasculitides, arterial dissection)
  - Acute tubular necrosis (hypotension, hypovolemia, myoglobinuria, contrast dye, medications)
  - Acute interstitial nephritis (medications)
  - Acute glomerulonephritis (GN)
- FE_{Na} is usually >1%.

Postrenal Azotemia

- Due to obstruction; usually involves both kidneys.
- Common etiologies: benign prostatic hyperplasia, prostate cancer, cervical cancer, nephrolithiasis, retroperitoneal fibrosis.

Key History

- **General:** weight gain/loss, anorexia

- **HEENT:** frequent sinusitis (Wegener's granulomatosis), recent URI (IgA nephropathy), pharyngitis (postinfectious GN)

- **Pulmonary:** hemoptysis (lupus, Wegener's, Goodpasture's, endocarditis)

- **Skin:** skin rash (vasculitis, drug reaction/interstitial nephritis)

- **GI:** vomiting, diarrhea (prerenal azotemia), bloody diarrhea (hemolytic uremic syndrome)

- **Genitourinary:** hematuria (GN, nephrolithiasis)

- **Medications:** NSAIDs, COX-2 inhibitors, ACE inhibitors, antibiotics (sulfa, penicillin, methicillin, nafcillin, cephalosporins), diuretics, IV contrast dye

- **Social history:** IV drug abuse

- **Medical history:**

  - HIV, sickle cell disease, endocarditis (focal segmental glomerulosclerosis)

  - Hepatitis (membranoproliferative GN)

  - Hodgkin's disease, lymphoproliferative disorder (minimal change disease)

  - Lupus (lupus GN)

Focused Physical Exam

- **Vital signs:** BP (orthostatics), heart rate, weight

- **Cardiovascular:** bruits (peripheral vascular disease), pulses, peripheral edema, murmurs

- **Skin:** malar rash (lupus), palpable purpura (leukocytoclastic vasculitis), drug rash, livedo reticularis (cholesterol emboli), peripheral stigmata of endocarditis (Roth spots, splinter hemorrhages, Osler's nodes)

- **Genitourinary:** prostate exam, pelvic exam (obstruction)

Evaluation

- **Labs:** electrolytes, CBC, UA with micro/macro (blood), urine sediment (casts), urine electrolytes (sodium), creatine kinase, albumin.

- **Renal U/S:** rule out parenchymal disease, obstruction; consider Doppler studies for renal artery stenosis.

- See Fig. 22-1 for algorithm for ARF evaluation.

Management

- Treatment is determined by the etiology.

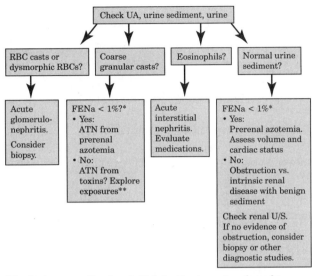

FIG. 22-1.
Algorithm for evaluation of acute renal failure.

* Avoid nephrotoxic agents.

* Treat hyperphosphatemia, hyperkalemia, and metabolic acidosis.

* Maintain a euvolemic state.

* For suspected glomerulonephritis, refer to a nephrologist for biopsy.

* Renal replacement therapy (i.e., dialysis) is indicated when

  * Hyperkalemia is refractory to medical management.

  * Acidosis is refractory to medical management.

  * There is evidence of gross volume overload (pulmonary edema).

  * There are symptoms of uremia (pericardial rub, altered mental status).

When to Refer

* Refer to a nephrologist for GN, ARF of unclear etiology (readily reversible), and chronic renal failure (CRF).

What to Tell the Patient

With prompt diagnosis and treatment, many causes of ARF are reversible, allowing many patients to return to their baseline renal function.

CHRONIC RENAL FAILURE
Definition and Etiology

- **CRF** is defined as a progressive decline in renal function; usually occurs at GFR <50 mL/min.

- **End-stage renal disease (ESRD)** is defined as the degree of renal failure that would cause the death of a patient unless some form of dialysis were performed.

- The most common causes of CRF in the United States are diabetes and HTN.

- Rarer causes: multiple myeloma, amyloidosis, polycystic kidney disease, lupus nephritis, obstructive uropathy, chronic NSAID use, and renovascular disease.

Key History

- **General:** generalized weakness, fatigue, pruritus

- **GI:** nausea, anorexia (uremia)

- **Pulmonary:** dyspnea (volume status)

- **Cardiovascular:** shortness of breath, paroxysmal nocturnal dyspnea, orthopnea, lower extremity edema (volume overload), chest pain (uremic pericarditis, ESRD increases risk of coronary artery disease)

- **Orthopedic:** generalized bone pain (hyperparathyroidism)

- **Skin:** "calciphylaxis" (calcified vessels, disposed to thrombosis, present as painful violaceous skin rash with ulceration and necrosis)

- **Medical history:** underlying etiology of CRF (see above)

- **Social history:** family support, patient compliance, lifestyle, location, IV drug use (suitability as a candidate for dialysis)

Focused Physical Exam

- **Vital signs:** BP (monitoring essential in CRF patients)

- **Cardiovascular:** rub (heard in uremic pericarditis), S_4 gallop (patients on dialysis may have left ventricular hypertrophy, diastolic dysfunction)

- **Pulmonary:** crackles

- **Skin:** calciphylaxis, edema, xanthelasmas, bullae (CRF, nephrotic syndrome)

Evaluation

- **Labs:** Chem 7, Ca^{2+}, phosphorus, Mg^{2+}, fasting lipid profile, 24-hr urine for protein and creatinine, parathyroid hormone (PTH) level, hepatitis panel
- **ECG**
- **Echocardiography:** in setting of pericarditis

Management

- **BP:** Goal in patients with CRF is <130/80 (will often require several agents).
- **Proteinuria:** Patients with CRF and proteinuria should be on an ACE inhibitor or angiotensin II receptor blocker; shown to decrease proteinuria and the progression to ESRD.
- **Acidosis:**
  - Correct acidosis, as it increases bone turnover and muscle catabolism.
  - Start bicarbonate therapy when bicarb level of <15 for patients not on hemodialysis. Starting dose: $NaHCO_3$, 650 mg PO tid, goal bicarb level >20.
- **Anemia:**
  - Anemia is a problem among patients with CRF (secondary to decreased erythropoietin production by kidney).
  - **Erythropoietin** should be initiated by a nephrologist when Hgb <10.
  - **Iron deficiency:** the most common cause of resistance to erythropoietin.
    - In CRF patient: defined as a ferritin <100, transferrin saturation <20%.
    - **IV iron therapy** is the preferred method of replacement in CRF.
  - Be sure to consider and exclude other causes of anemia (see Chap. 14, Hematology).
- **Hyperparathyroidism:**
  - Check PTH levels in patients with CRF (GFR <50 mL/min); goal PTH in these patients is around 100.

- Treatment includes:
  - Phosphorus dietary restriction.
  - Calculate Ca^{2+}-phosphate product: $[Ca^{2+}] \times [PO_4^{2-}]$
  - If calcium phosphate product <50, initiate treatment with calcium salts, such as Ca carbonate, Ca acetate, and Ca citrate; Ca carbonate is preferred (better tolerated than Ca acetate). Starting dose: Ca carbonate, 500 mg PO tid with meals.
  - If hypercalcemia or Ca^{2+}-phosphate product ≥50, then start noncalcium phosphate binder, such as sevalemer (Renagel), 800 mg PO tid.
  - Goal: Ca^{2+}-phosphate product <50.
  - Vitamin D supplementation.
- Indications for parathyroidectomy:
  - Hyperparathyroidism no longer responsive to medical therapy
  - Calciphylaxis
  - Hypercalcemia
  - Metastatic calcifications
  - Renal transplant candidates
- **Dialysis:** Decision to begin dialysis is made in conjunction with a nephrologist.
- **Renal transplantation:** Definitive long-term management for ESRD.

When to Refer

Refer all patients with CRF (GFR <50 mL/min) to a nephrologist.

What to Tell the Patient

- Patients should understand the importance of good BP and blood sugar control in preventing the progression of their renal disease.
- Initiating dialysis (hemodialysis or peritoneal dialysis) is a major lifestyle change for patients and their families. It requires much dedication and compliance.

HEMATURIA
Definition

- The presence of RBC in the urine. It can be macroscopic (gross) or microscopic.

- Hematuria carries a broad differential diagnosis and can be divided into glomerular and nonglomerular causes (Table 22-1).

Key History

- **General:** duration, amount of hematuria; fevers (autoimmune disease or endocarditis); weight loss (malignancy); recent trauma; exercise habits (jogging, bicycling)

- **Pulmonary:** hemoptysis (Goodpasture's disease, Wegener's granulomatosis, lupus, vasculitis)

- **Genitourinary:**

    - Urinary frequency, urgency, dysuria, flank pain (UTI/pyelonephritis)

    - Urinary hesitancy, weak stream, and postvoid dribbling (bladder outlet obstruction)

    - Colicky flank pain radiating to the groin (nephro- or urolithiasis), urethral discharge (urethritis)

- **Musculoskeletal:** arthralgias or arthritis (autoimmune causes, such as SLE)

- **Skin:** rash (systemic vasculitis or lupus)

- **Hematologic:** blood transfusions, risk factors for HIV, hepatitis B and C

- **Medical history:**

    - Recent pharyngitis (postinfectious GN)

    - Recent mucosal infection, such as URI, UTI, enteritis, etc. (Henoch-Schönlein purpura, IgA nephropathy)

    - Bloody diarrhea (hemolytic-uremic syndrome)

    - Recurrent sinusitis/otitis (Wegener's)

    - Sickle cell disease

- **Medications:** anticoagulants, such as coumadin, heparin (predisposition to bleeding); cyclophosphamide (hemorrhagic cystitis, bladder cancer)

- **Social history:** IV drug use (IV heroin, HIV associated with focal segmental glomerulosclerosis), other risk factors for HIV, hepatitis, and endocarditis

- **Sexual history:** HIV risk factors, hepatitis, chlamydia, and gonorrhea; menstrual history important in women

TABLE 22-1.
CAUSES OF HEMATURIA

Glomerular
  Proliferative GN
    IgA nephropathy
    Postinfectious GN
    Crescentic GN
    Membranoproliferative GN
    SLE
    Systemic vasculitis
    Chronic bacteremia
    Mixed cryoglobulinemia
  Nonproliferative GN
    Minimal change disease
    Focal glomerulosclerosis
    Membranous nephropathy
    Hemolytic uremic syndrome
  Familial glomerular disease
    Alport syndrome
    Familial benign hematuria
    Fabry disease
    Nail-patella syndrome
Nonglomerular
  Non–urinary tract
    Menstrual bleeding
    Vaginitis
    Foreign body
    Anal fissure/rectal bleed
  Vascular
    Renal vein thrombosis
    Renal infarction
    Malignant HTN
    AV malformation

Infections
  Acute cystitis
  Prostatitis
  Urethritis
  TB
Papillary necrosis
  Analgesic abuse
  Sickle cell disease
  Diabetes
  Obstructive uropathy
  Alcoholism
Calculi
  Renal
  Ureteral
  Bladder
  Prostatic
Drugs
  Cyclophosphamide (hemor-
    rhagic cystitis)
  Acute interstitial nephritis
  Heparin
  Coumadin
Familial
  Polycystic kidney disease
  Medullary cystic disease
  Medullary sponge kidney
Trauma
  Renal contusion/laceration
  Bladder trauma (exercise)
  Bladder decompression
  Foreign body
Neoplasms
  Renal cell cancer
  Transitional cell cancer
  Prostate carcinoma
  Urethral squamous cell cancer

GN, glomerulonephritis.
Adapted from Greenberg A. *Primer of kidney diseases*, 2nd ed. San Diego:
Academic Press/National Kidney Foundation, 1998.

- **Family history:**
  - Hematuria without consequence (benign familial hematuria)
  - Deafness and kidney disease (Alport's disease)
  - Cerebral aneurysms and kidney disease (autosomal-dominant polycystic kidney disease)
  - Hypercalcemia/nephrolithiasis

Focused Physical Exam

- **Vital signs:** HTN (nephritis); calculate BMI (obesity is a risk factor for focal segmental glomerulosclerosis)
- **HEENT:** evidence of sinusitis/otitis or pharyngitis, nasal bridge destruction (Wegener's granulomatosis), periorbital edema (glomerular etiology with proteinuria), Roth spots (endocarditis)
- **Neck:** bruits, thyroid nodules (multiple endocrine neoplasia)
- **Cardiovascular:** murmurs (endocarditis)
- **Pulmonary:** abnormal lung sounds (vasculitis)
- **Abdominal:** hepatosplenomegaly, ascites, stigmata of liver disease (hepatitis), masses (urinary tract malignancies)
- **Extremities:** peripheral edema; splinter hemorrhages, Osler nodes, and Janeway lesions (endocarditis); arthritis (lupus, cryoglobulinemia)
- **Skin:** rashes (vasculitis), palpable purpura (Henoch-Schönlein purpura, especially if purpura is on lower extremities)
- **Genitourinary:** prostate exam (prostatis/prostate carcinoma)
- **Lymph:** lymphadenopathy (malignancy)

Evaluation

Labs

- Chem 7, CBC, UA with sedimentation, calcium level, uric acid level.
  - RBC casts and dysmorphic RBCs on UA suggest a glomerular origin of hematuria (increased serum Cr, proteinuria, HTN also suggestive).
  - You should always spin your own urine: don't count on the lab to find casts for you.
- If clinically indicated (RBC casts or dysmorphic RBCs): ANA, ANCA, HIV, hepatitis panel, anti-GBM, anti-*Streptolysin O* antibodies, blood cultures, and cryoglobulins.

- **Urine cytology** is necessary in patients >50 or in whom malignancy is a possibility.

- **24-hr creatinine collection** to estimate creatinine clearance and proteinuria can also be helpful.

Radiology

- **Chest x-ray** if pulmonary findings in history or on exam

- **Chest CT** if suspicious for Wegener's or Goodpasture's

- **Abdominal CT scan, renal U/S** to evaluate for stones, hydronephrosis, renal cysts, renal malignancy

- **Cystoscopy** evaluation of bladder for bladder mass

Echocardiography

- If endocarditis is suspected, a TEE is the diagnostic procedure of choice.

Diagnosis

See Figure 22-2.

Management

Management of specific conditions is beyond the scope of this discussion, but:

- Important to note: In cases in which patients have rapidly declining renal function, it is imperative to refer patients to specialists (nephrologists, urologists, or oncologists) as soon as possible.

- The longer the delay in evaluation and treatment, the more likely irreversible damage and permanent sequelae will result.

When to Refer

- Patients with suspected or known GN (immediate nephrology referral).

- All patients with stones (urology, possibly to nephrology). Often, no intervention will be performed; however, it is important for such patients to have regular follow-up.

- Any patient with newly diagnosed malignancy of the urinary tract (urology, oncology).

What to Tell the Patient

- Hematuria has many benign causes (as well as more serious ones).

- Patients are often very apprehensive about hematuria; assure the patient that you will perform a thorough evaluation.

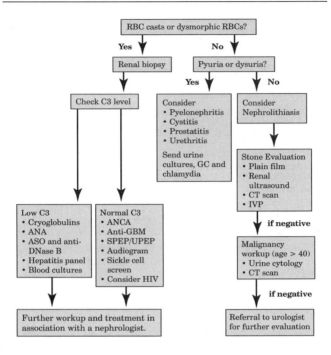

FIG. 22-2.
Diagnostic approach to hematuria patients. ANCA, antineutrophil cytoplasmic antibodies; ASO, antistreptolysin-O; FHx, family history; Hx, history; IVP, IV pyelogram; PMH, past medical history; SPEP/UPEP, serum protein electrophoresis/urine protein electrophoresis. (Adapted from Greenberg A. *Primer on kidney diseases,* 2nd ed. San Diego: Academic Press/National Kidney Foundation, 1998.)

PROTEINURIA

Definitions

- **Proteinuria:** >300 mg of albumin excreted in a 24-hr period (normal: <30 mg/24 hrs)

- **Nephrotic range proteinuria:** >3.5 g of protein excreted/day. Nephrotic syndrome consists of nephrotic range proteinuria, hypoalbuminemia, edema, and dyslipidemia.

- **Microalbuminuria:** Protein excretion of 30–300 mg/day.

Etiology

- **Overflow proteinuria:** myeloma (suspect in patients who have large amounts of protein in urine and negative dipstick)

- **Tubulointerstitial disease**
- **Glomerular proteinuria:**
  - Functional proteinuria: transient proteinuria after exercise, fever, congestive heart failure
  - Orthostatic proteinuria
- **Nephrotic syndrome:**
  - **Diabetes**
  - **Minimal change disease:** associated with recent viral illness, allergy, atopy, NSAID use, Hodgkin's disease
  - **Focal segmental glomerulosclerosis:** associated with HIV, heroin use, African-American race, and obesity
  - **Membranous glomerulopathy:** most common cause of primary nephrotic syndrome in adults; associated with a variety of causes, including drugs (NSAIDs, gold, penicillamine, captopril), hepatitis B and C, malignancy, and lupus nephritis
  - **Membranoproliferative glomerulonephritis:** typically causes a nephritic picture but can also produce the nephrotic syndrome, associated with hepatitis C and cryoglobulinemia
  - **Amyloidosis:** associated with plasma cell dyscrasias (multiple myeloma) and chronic inflammatory processes (rheumatoid arthritis, osteomyelitis, chronic tuberculosis infection)

Key History

- **General:** weight loss (malignancy), fevers, and night sweats (malignancy, TB)
- **HEENT:** periorbital edema (nephrotic syndrome)
- **Cardiovascular:** CHF symptoms (volume overload)
- **Skin:** rashes (vasculitis)
- **Endocrine:** polyuria, polydipsia, weight gain (diabetes)
- **Social history:** IV drug abuse, heroin use (focal segmental glomerulosclerosis)

Focused Physical Exam

- **Vital signs:** BP (HTN), BMI (obesity)
- **HEENT:** periorbital edema, xanthelasma (hyperlipidemia)
- **Cardiovascular:** peripheral edema, gallops
- **Skin:** rashes

- **Extremities:** xanthomas (lipid nodules in tendon)

Evaluation

- **Lab data:** Chem 7, CBC, UA with micro/macro, 24-hr urine collection for protein and creatinine. If indicated, HIV, hepatitis B/C, cryoglobulins, lipids (nephrotic syndrome).

- **Spot urine protein/creatinine ratio:** can be used to estimate protein excretion but should not be a substitute for 24-hr urine sample. *Never quantify proteinuria in the setting of an acute febrile illness or heart failure exacerbation.*

- **Microalbuminuria:**

  - Screening for microalbuminuria is very important, as it is a predictor of overt proteinuria, renal failure, and cardiovascular mortality.

  - Can do 24-hr urine sample or spot urine sample for albumin/creatinine ratio.

  - Should be done yearly in diabetics.

- For algorithm describing proteinuria evaluation, see Fig. 22-3.

Treatment

- Ultimately, treating the underlying cause effectively can often lead to a reversal of the proteinuria.

- **Orthostatic proteinuria** does not require treatment.

- **ACE inhibitors:** decrease intraglomerular pressure and thus decrease proteinuria. Have been shown to decrease the progression towards overt proteinuria and renal failure in diabetic patients.

- **Lipid reduction:** in patients with nephrotic syndrome, may improve with decreased proteinuria. Consider lipid reduction therapy with a statin.

- **BP control:** goal BP is <130/80 in proteinuria patients. ACE inhibitor is first-line therapy.

- **Diuretics:** to control edema; loop diuretics may not be as efficacious in this setting because they are protein bound.

What to Tell the Patient

- Orthostatic proteinuria is a benign condition, and patients should not worry that they have diseased kidneys.

- For diabetics, tight glucose and BP control will help prevent the progression to overt renal disease.

- Proteinuria is an independent risk factor for cardiovascular mortality and overt renal failure, so patients should be monitored closely.

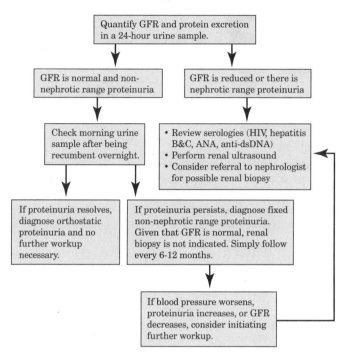

FIG. 22-3.
Algorithm for the evaluation of proteinuria.

When to Refer

Refer to nephrologist for nephrotic range proteinuria, proteinuria with decreased GFR, or hematuria.

SUGGESTED READING

Greenberg A. *Primer on kidney diseases.* San Diego: Academic Press/National Kidney Foundation, 1998.

Johnson RJ, Feehally J. *Comprehensive clinical nephrology.* St. Louis: Mosby, 2000.

23 Women's Health

It's not that time of the month!

AMENORRHEA

Definitions

- **Primary amenorrhea:** Failure to menstruate by 16 yrs with secondary sexual characteristics or failure to menstruate by 14 yrs with absence of secondary sexual characteristics.
- **Secondary amenorrhea:** Absence of menses for 6 mos or for three consecutive menstrual cycles.

Differential Diagnosis

- **Hypothalamic disorders:** hypothyroidism, excessive exercise, anorexia/bulimia, weight loss, stress, anovulation, chronic diseases, craniopharyngioma, Kallman's syndrome, post-pill amenorrhea
- **Anterior pituitary disorders:** pituitary adenoma (prolactinoma), lymphocytic hypophysitis, Sheehan's syndrome, TB, sarcoidosis, carotid artery aneurysm, dermoid cyst, pituitary ablation
- **Ovarian disorders:** infection (mumps), autoimmune disease, chemotherapy, radiation, gonadal dysgenesis, iatrogenic (surgical), polycystic ovary syndrome
- **Uterine/outflow tract disorders:** Asherman's syndrome, androgen insensitivity, müllerian anomalies/agenesis, true hermaphrodites

Key History

- **General:** cold intolerance, weight loss, night sweats
- **HEENT:** headache, visual changes (pituitary disorder), dental caries (bulimia)
- **Breast:** galactorrhea (prolactinoma)
- **Medical history:** hypothyroidism, mumps, autoimmune disease, malignancy (radiation, chemo), tuberculosis, anorexia/bulimia
- **Gynecologic:** number of pregnancies, hypotension during pregnancy (Sheehan's syndrome), age of onset of menses, length of menstrual cycles, onset of amenorrhea, birth control method, gynecologic surgery, dissection and curettage
- **Medications:** oral contraceptives, chemotherapy
- **Social history:** diet, exercise/sports participation (excessive)

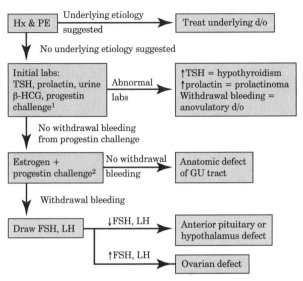

FIG. 23-1.
Algorithm for evaluation of amenorrhea. Hx, history.
[1]Progestin challenge: medroxyprogesterone acetate, 5 mg PO qd ×10 days.
[2]Estrogen + progestin challenge: estradiol, 2 mg PO qd ×21 days + medroxyprogesterone acetate, 5 mg PO qd ×10 days.

Focused Physical Exam

- **Vital signs:** weight (document)

- **HEENT:** dental caries (bulimia), thyroid, visual fields (pituitary adenoma)

- **Breast:** galactorrhea (prolactinoma)

- **Genitourinary:** ovarian abnormalities, uterus (present/absent)

- **Skin:** chafing (bulimia), acanthosis nigricans, hirsutism

Evaluation

See Fig. 23-1.

Management

- Amenorrhea management depends on the specific etiology.

  - **Hypothyroidism** treatment requires replacement of thyroid hormone. See Chap. 10, Endocrinology.

  - **Post-pill amenorrhea** is common after hormonal contraception. Patients on oral contraceptive pills may require 6 mos for the return of menstrual function. For patients on depot medroxyprogesterone acetate (MPA), it may require up to 1 yr for return of menses.

- **Other hypothalamic disorders** include anorexia, bulimia, stress, and excessive exercise, all of which decrease GnRH secretion. Patients with prolonged hypothalamic amenorrhea require hormone replacement therapy (HRT) (see below).

- **Pituitary adenomas,** such as prolactinomas, require further workup with an MRI of the brain. Medical and surgical treatment options exist.

- **Ovarian disorders** result in chronic amenorrhea and require HRT.

- **Asherman's syndrome** results from the development of multiple intrauterine synechiae after uterine curettage or infection. Diagnosis is by hysteroscopy or hysterosalpingogram. Treatment is by hysteroscopic adhesiolysis and estrogen.

- Patients with **chronic amenorrhea** should be placed on HRT to prevent bone loss and vaginal atrophy:

  - HRT: Conjugated estrogen, 0.625 mg PO qd + medroxyprogesterone, 5 mg PO qd for 2 wks/mo.

  - Oral contraceptives are also appropriate.

- Patients who desire pregnancy may be candidates for ovulation induction.

When to Refer

- Refer to gynecologist if the diagnosis is not clear or if the patient desires pregnancy.

- Patients with anorexia or bulimia require counseling and referral to a psychiatrist.

What to Tell the Patient

- Patients with chronic amenorrhea may need HRT to prevent bone loss and vaginal atrophy.

- Patients with amenorrhea still may be able to get pregnant, depending on etiology.

CONTRACEPTION
Barrier Methods

See Table 23-1.

Hormonal Methods

See Table 23-2 and Table 23-3.

**TABLE 23-1.
BARRIER CONTRACEPTION METHODS**

Method	Failure rate (%)	Notes
Condom	14	Made of latex, silicone, polyurethane, or lamb intestine.
		Should be placed before intercourse and removed after sex.
		Contraindications: Avoid latex condoms in latex-allergic patients; avoid oil-based lubricants.
Female condom	21	Made of polyurethane.
		Can be inserted up to 8 hrs before intercourse.
		Increases risk of UTI.
Diaphragm	18–20	Must be fitted by physician.
		Can be used in combination with spermicides to reduce failure rate.
		Should be placed 6 hrs before intercourse and left in place 6–24 hrs after.
Cervical cap	18–20	Must be fitted by physician.
		Can be used in combination with spermicides to reduce failure rate.
		Should be left in place for 8 hrs after coitus.
Spermicides	20–25	Tablets and suppositories last 1 hr.
		Creams and foams last 8 hrs.
		Can be used in combination with condoms, diaphragm, and cervical cap.
IUD	0.1–2	ParaGuard (copper) is approved for 10 yrs; Progestasert (progestin) is approved for 1 yr.
		Contraindications: pregnancy, pelvic malignancy, undiagnosed vaginal bleeding, high-risk STD behavior, immunosuppression, abnormal Pap smear, history of ectopic pregnancy.
		Risks of IUD placement: infection, displacement, ectopic pregnancy.
		No long-term effects on fertility.

TABLE 23-2.
HORMONAL CONTRACEPTION METHODS

Depo-Provera (medroxyprogesterone acetate)

- Failure rate: 0.30%

- Dosage: 150 mg IM q3mos. Should be given within 7 days of the last menstrual cycle; otherwise, a backup method is required.

- Contraindications: pregnancy, unexplained vaginal bleeding, coagulation disorder, liver abnormalities, severe cardiovascular disease, severe depression.

- Side effects: irregular menstrual bleeding, breast tenderness, weight gain, depression.

- No long-term effects on fertility; however, delay in conception up to 9 mos can occur after discontinuation.

Lunelle (medroxyprogesterone acetate + estradiol)

- Failure rate: 0.1–0.4%

- Dosage: 25 mg medroxyprogesterone/5 mg estradiol IM q28 days.

- Contraindications: See oral contraceptive contraindications.

- Side effects: depression, anxiety, weight gain, mood lability.

Norplant (levonorgestrel)

- Failure rate: 0.05%

- Implanted in upper arm; effective for up to 5 yrs.

- Backup contraception should be used for first 3 days.

- Contraindications: thromboembolic disease, undiagnosed vaginal bleeding, liver disease, breast cancer, pregnancy.

- Side effects: breakthrough bleeding, ectopic pregnancy, weight gain, mastalgia, headache, galactorrhea, acne, ovarian cysts.

- No long-term effects on fertility.

Oral contraceptives

Combination

- Failure rate: 0.1–3%

- Available in a variety of dosages and formulations, including a weekly patch.

- Low-dose pills contain <50 µg of estradiol/pill.

- Monophasic formulations contain the same amount of hormone in each pill; triphasic formulations contain variable amounts of estrogen and progesterone.

- Contraindications: DVT, thrombophlebitis, impaired liver function, breast cancer, undiagnosed vaginal bleeding, pregnancy, smokers >age 35, previous MI/stroke, significant CAD.

(*continued*)

**TABLE 23-2.
CONTINUED**

- Benefits: decreased risk of endometrial and ovarian cancer, decreased acne.

- Risks: increased risk of DVT, breast cancer, cholelithiasis, liver adenomas, HTN.

- Side effects: breakthrough bleeding, amenorrhea, nausea, weight gain (average 5–7 lbs), breast tenderness, headaches. Can exacerbate migraine headaches, HTN, and SLE; can increase triglycerides.

- Drug interactions: decreased efficacy with anticonvulsants and antibiotics. *Advise patients to use backup contraception while taking antibiotics.*

- No long-term effects on fertility; however, delay in conception up to several months can occur after discontinuation.

Progestin only

- Option for patients in whom combination OCPs are contraindicated.

- Effects of the pill last only 24 hrs; pill must be taken at the same time every day.

- Pill should be started on the first day of cycle and backup method used for 7 days.

- Contraindications: pregnancy, breast cancer, liver disease, undiagnosed vaginal bleeding, CAD.

- Side effects: nausea, vomiting, bloating, amenorrhea, breakthrough bleeding, edema, breast tenderness, weight gain, headache, acne.

- Drug interactions: decreased efficacy with antibiotics. *Advise patients to use backup contraception while taking antibiotics.*

- No long-term effects on fertility.

Emergency contraception

- Appropriate discussion regarding other contraceptive methods should be addressed in follow-up.

Combination OCPs

- Need to take 100 µg of ethinyl estradiol (of any OCP) + 0.50 mg levonorgestrel within 72 hrs of intercourse.

- Preven: Prepackaged kit; take 2 and repeat 2 pills in 12 hrs.

- Side effects: Severe nausea and vomiting; may need to prescribe concomitant antiemetic. Otherwise, same side effects as OCPs above.

- Contraindications: Same as for OCPs.

Progestin-only OCPs

- Need to take 1.5 mg levonorgestrel within 72 hrs of intercourse.

- Plan B: Prepackaged kit; take 2 pills 12 hrs apart.

CAD, coronary artery disease; DVT, deep venous thrombosis; OCP, oral contraceptive pill.

TABLE 23-3.
RECOMMENDATIONS FOR MISSED PILLS

Pills missed	Recommendation	Backup contraception needed?
1	Take pill ASAP	No
2 (in wks 1 or 2)	Take 2 pills daily ×2 days	Yes, for 7 days
2 (in wk 3) or >3	Start new pill pack	Yes, for 7 days

ABNORMAL UTERINE BLEEDING
Definitions

- **Menorrhagia:** prolonged (>7 days) or heavy (>80 mL) menses

- **Metrorrhagia:** irregular bleeding

- **Menometrorrhagia:** prolonged or heavy menses with irregular bleeding

- **Polymenorrhea:** menses at intervals <21 days

- **Oligomenorrhea:** menses at intervals >35 days

- **Dysfunctional uterine bleeding (DUB):** The most common cause of abnormal uterine bleeding in adolescents and perimenopausal women. DUB is a diagnosis of exclusion. >90% of patients with DUB are anovulatory; the remainder are ovulatory.

Differential Diagnosis
Organic Causes

- Pregnancy complications (abortion, ectopic pregnancy, molar pregnancy)

- Malignancy (cervical, endometrial, ovarian, vulvar, vaginal)

- Infection (PID, cervicitis, vulvovaginitis)

- Trauma

- Foreign body

- Polyps (cervical, endometrial)

- Leiomyomas

- Adenomyosis

Systemic Diseases

- Coagulopathy

- Liver disease

- Thyroid disease

Dysfunctional Uterine Bleeding

- Anovulatory (eating disorder, exercise, polycystic ovarian syndrome [PCOS], obesity, androgen excess)

- Ovulatory

- See Table 23-4 for breakdown by age group.

Key History

- **General:** heat/cold intolerance, dry skin, weight loss/gain (thyroid disease); obesity, hirsutism (PCOS)

- **Gynecologic:** menstrual history (age at menarche, amount, duration, pain), menstrual calendar (pad counts), basal body temperature chart (evaluate ovulation), genital trauma, sexual history (possibility of pregnancy)

- **Medical history:** thyroid disease, gynecologic cancer, PCOS, bleeding disorder

- **Medications:** exogenous hormones

Focused Physical Exam

- **Abdominal:** hepatomegaly (liver disease)

- **Gynecologic:** pelvic exam, speculum exam, cervical/vaginal lesions, leiomyomas

- **Rectal:** hemorrhoids, anal fissures, guaiac stool

Evaluation

- **Labs:** CBC with platelets, TSH, ferritin, PT/PTT, bleeding time, LFTs, UA (hematuria).

- **Urine beta-hCG** (rule out pregnancy).

- **Pap smear.**

- **Cervical cultures** to rule out infections (*Chlamydia, Gonorrhea*).

- **Endometrial sampling** or endocervical curettage (if >35 yrs) to rule out endometrial hyperplasia or cancer.

- Consider referring to gynecology for a vaginal U/S or hysteroscopy to look for polyps, endometrial hyperplasia, and myomas.

Management

Management depends on the underlying etiology.

TABLE 23-4.
DIFFERENTIAL DIAGNOSIS OF ABNORMAL
UTERINE BLEEDING BY AGE GROUP

Prepubertal	Adolescent	Reproductive	Perimenopausal	Postmenopausal
Vulvovaginitis	Anovulation	Pregnancy	Anovulation	Endometrial lesions
Foreign body	Pregnancy	Anovulation	Leiomyomas	Exogenous hormones
Precocious puberty	Exogenous hormones	Leiomyomas	Polyps	Atrophic vaginitis
Neoplasms	Coagulopathy	Thyroid disease	Thyroid disease	Other neoplasm

Adapted from Berek JS, Adaski EY, Hillard PA, eds. *Novak's gynecology*, 12th ed. Philadelphia: Lippincott Williams & Wilkins, 1996.

Medical Management

- **Estrogens:** Conjugated estrogen, 2.5–5 mg PO q6h × 21–25 days. Add MPA, 10 mg PO qd for the last 7 days (to induce withdrawal bleeding).

- **Progestins:**
  - MPA, 10 mg qd for 10 days/mo
  - Depot MPA, 150 mg IM q1–3mos
  - Progesterone IUD

- **Oral contraceptive pills**
  - **Progestin or combination oral contraceptive pills** are the long-term treatment of choice for DUB.

- **NSAIDs** decrease menstrual cramping and bleeding: ibuprofen, 600–800 mg PO q8h, or naproxen, 250–500 mg PO q12h.

Surgical Options

- **Dilation and curettage** provides immediate relief, but long-term therapy is usually required.

- **Endometrial ablation** is used in patients with DUB without genital tract pathology. Improvement has been noted in >90% of patients.

- **Hysterectomy** provides definitive therapy.

When to Refer

Refer to gynecologist for bleeding that does not respond to treatment, suspected cancer, or surgical treatment.

DYSMENORRHEA
Definition

- Cyclic lower abdominal cramping at the time of menses.

- **Primary dysmenorrhea** results from prostaglandin release at the time of menses and occurs in the absence of pelvic pathology. Onset is typically shortly after menarche.

- **Secondary dysmenorrhea** occurs when there is pelvic pathology and can occur at any time in life.

- **Causes of secondary dysmenorrhea:**
  - Cervical stenosis
  - Adenomyosis
  - Imperforate hymen
  - Ovarian remnant syndrome

- Transverse vaginal septum
- Pelvic congestion
- Endometriosis
- Leiomyomas

Key History

- **GI:** cramping, abdominal pain before or at onset of menses, nausea, diarrhea
- **Gynecologic:** menstrual history (age at menarche, duration, flow)

Focused Physical Exam

Gynecologic: uterine tenderness, nodularity in vaginal cul-de-sac, adnexal mass (endometriosis), leiomyomas, anatomic abnormalities (cervical stenosis, imperforate hymen)

Evaluation

History and physical exam are generally sufficient for diagnosis.

Management

- **Medications** are the mainstay of treatment for primary dysmenorrhea.
  - **NSAIDs** are the treatment of choice. During menses, NSAIDs should be taken on a scheduled basis. Ibuprofen, 600–800 mg PO q8h, naproxen (Naprosyn, Aleve), 250–500 mg PO bid, or can also use COX-2 inhibitors (rofecoxib, 50 mg PO qd)
- **Oral contraceptive pills** often relieve the pain of dysmenorrhea and should be considered if birth control is also desired.

Treatment for secondary dysmenorrhea is based on the underlying etiology.

When to Refer

Refer to a gynecologist for pain unresponsive to treatment or for evaluation for secondary dysmenorrhea.

What to Tell the Patient

Dysmenorrhea is usually benign, and only symptomatic treatment is necessary.

MENOPAUSE AND HORMONE REPLACEMENT THERAPY
Definition

- Menopause has occurred when menstrual periods cease for 1 yr.

- It can be physiologic, caused by the cessation of ovarian follicular development, or secondary to surgical removal of the ovaries or the uterus.
- The average age of menopause is around 50, but women from their late 30s to late 50s can experience it.

Differential Diagnosis

Consider for younger patients and those who have atypical symptoms:

- Hypothyroidism
- Pituitary dysfunction
- Ovarian dysfunction
- Adrenal dysfunction
- PCOS
- Pregnancy
- Asherman's syndrome (adhesion of the uterus that prevents menstrual blood flow)

Key History

- **General:** hot flashes, night sweats, fatigue, headaches
- **Genitourinary:** irregular menstrual cycles, amenorrhea, burning/ itching of vagina, dyspareunia
- **Psychiatric:** depression, anxiety, insomnia, nervousness, irritability, difficulty with concentration
- **Sexual:** decreased libido, birth control, possibility of pregnancy
- **Medical history:** breast cancer, BRCA1 or BRCA2 genes, hypercoagulable state, liver disease, endometrial cancer
- **Family history:** mother's age at menopause (may correlate), breast cancer, ovarian cancer
- **Social history:** smoking (tends to promote early menopause), alcohol use

Focused Physical Exam

- **Vital signs:** BP, heart rate
- **Cardiovascular:** rate, rhythm, murmurs
- **Breast:** abnormal lumps
- **Genitourinary:** vaginal atrophy, lesions

Evaluation

- If the patient has typical symptoms of menopause and is in the right age group, no further workup is necessary.

- Consider **urine or serum beta-hCG** to rule out pregnancy before starting hormone therapy.

- **Labs:** FSH (elevated), estrogen (decreased). Consider LH level if ruling out PCOS (LH:FSH typically 2:1).

- To **rule out other causes** of menopausal symptoms:

  - TSH (elevated in hypothyroidism)

  - Prolactin level (elevated in prolactinoma)

  - Corticotropin stimulation test (cortisol lower than normal in adrenal insufficiency)

  - MRI to rule out pituitary pathology (if suspected)

- **Pap smear.**

- Consider **endometrial biopsy** in a patient with irregular menstrual bleeding or postmenopausal bleeding.

- **Mammogram** (before starting HRT).

Management

The issue: HRT vs no HRT.

- Data from recent trials suggest that, for most women, the risks of combination long-term HRT may outweigh the benefits. Current recommendations are that HRT should be prescribed only for temporary relief.

- The Women's Health Initiative (WHI) study showed a higher risk of coronary disease, stroke, pulmonary embolism, and invasive breast cancer after 5 yrs, and possibly dementia after 4 yrs, for women taking estrogen and progesterone.

- The Heart and Estrogen/Progestin Replacement studies (HERS and HERS II) demonstrated no benefit to using estrogen with progesterone for secondary prevention of heart disease in women. In fact, there was an *increased* risk of cardiovascular events in the first year after initiating HRT (this risk subsequently declined during follow-up).

- In addition, the HERS II trial demonstrated an increased risk of thromboembolic events (deep venous thrombosis/pulmonary embolism) and an increase in biliary tract surgery with estrogen and progesterone therapy.

- However, both the WHI and HERS II suggest that long-term HRT may decrease the risk of colon cancer and prevent bone fractures.

- See Table 23-5 for a summary of the risks and benefits of HRT.

- Figure 23-2 provides a decision-making algorithm for HRT use. Treatment decisions should be made on an individual basis, weighing risks, benefits, and patient preference.

Absolute contraindications to HRT:

- Unexplained vaginal bleeding
- Active liver disease
- History of venous thromboembolism or hypercoagulable state
- History of endometrial cancer
- History of breast cancer

Relative contraindications to HRT:

- Hypertriglyceridemia (decreased risk with transdermal estrogen)
- Active gallbladder disease
- Coronary artery disease
- Family history of breast cancer or carrier of BRCA1 or BRCA2 gene

Indications for HRT:

- Menopausal symptom relief (short-term use)
- Osteopenia, osteoporosis, or high risk for osteoporosis
- Table 23-5 summarizes benefits and risks of HRT.
- Figure 23-2 provides a decision-making algorithm for use of HRT.

TABLE 23-5.
BENEFITS AND RISKS OF COMBINATION HORMONE REPLACEMENT THERAPY

Benefits	Risks
Symptom relief	Increased risk of thromboembolic events (3× baseline)
Prevention of osteoporosis (decreases risk of vertebral fractures by 50%, hip fractures by 30%)	Increased risk of endometrial cancer with unopposed estrogen
? Reduction in risk of colorectal cancer (needs further study)	Increase in cardiovascular events and mortality in patients with coronary artery disease (within first year)
	Elevated triglycerides
	Increased risk of gallbladder disease (2–3× baseline)
	Possible increased risk of dementia (2× baseline) and urinary incontinence
	Increased risk of breast cancer

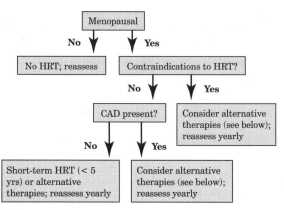

FIG. 23-2.
Decision-making algorithm for hormone replacement therapy. CAD, coronary artery disease. (Adapted from Manson JE, Martin KA. Postmenopausal hormone replacement therapy. *N Engl J Med* 2001;345:39.)

Prescribing HRT

- **Women with a uterus** must take both estrogen and progesterone for prevention of endometrial cancer. Typical prescribed regimens:

  - Estrogen, 0.625 mg and progesterone, 2.5 mg combinations, 1 pill PO qd

  - Estrogen, 0.625 mg PO qd + progesterone, 2.5 mg PO qd or 5–10 mg PO qd on days 1–10

  - Estradiol, 1–2 mg PO qd + progesterone as above

  - Transdermal estradiol, 50–100 µg qd + progesterone as above

- **Women status-post hysterectomy** can be prescribed estrogen only in the same dosages as above.

- **Side Effects**

  - Breast tenderness, breakthrough bleeding, monthly withdrawal bleeding (if on cyclic progesterone regimen), nausea, bloating, abdominal cramps, weight gain, headache (particularly exacerbation of migraine headaches), depression.

  - Studies are ongoing to determine the minimum amount of estrogen necessary for benefit. Consider decreasing dose if the patient does not tolerate the higher dose. Also, consider raising the dose as necessary to relieve symptoms (but may also increase risk of side effects).

- **Vaginal estrogen cream and/or vaginal lubricants** may be helpful for those with vaginal dryness or atrophy.

Monitoring

- Women should have **clinical breast exams, mammograms, pelvic exams,** and **Pap smears** q yr.
- **Irregular bleeding** requires referral to a gynecologist for evaluation for endometrial cancer.

Alternatives

- For **osteoporosis** treatment, see Chap. 10, Endocrinology.
- For **vasomotor symptoms:**
  - Avoidance of caffeine, alcohol, and spicy foods.
  - **Clonidine (Catapres),** 0.05–0.15 mg PO qd. Side effects: dry mouth, dizziness, sedation, nausea, headache, dry eyes, rebound HTN.
  - **Depo-Provera,** 150 mg IM q mo. Side effects: weight gain, nausea, hirsutism, breast tenderness, rash, acne.
  - **Soy products and black cohosh** have been shown to relieve some menopausal symptoms. However, these products also carry an increased risk of thromboembolism.
  - **SSRIs** may also be useful, particularly if underlying depression is present.

When to Refer

Refer to a gynecologist for difficult-to-control symptoms or irregular bleeding or if you do not feel comfortable managing HRT.

What to Tell the Patient

- Menopause is physiologic, and its symptoms can be treated.
- Counsel women on the risks and benefits of HRT. Recent trials have shown that for most women, the risks of long-term combination HRT (>5 yrs) may outweigh the benefits. However, short-term use (<5 yrs) may be beneficial to ameliorate symptoms and prevent fractures.
- Any postmenopausal bleeding or new breast lumps should be evaluated immediately.
- Ongoing studies are further examining the benefits and risks of estrogen:
  - Most recent data suggest that there is an elevated risk of heart disease, stroke, thrombosis, breast cancer, and gallbladder disease.
  - Benefits include symptom relief, reduction in bone fractures, and a possible reduction in colorectal cancer.

VAGINAL DISCHARGE
Key History

- **Genitourinary:**

  - Characterization of vaginal discharge: watery, "cottage cheese," frothy, purulent

  - Odor

  - Dyspareunia

  - Pruritus

  - History of new soap/detergent/feminine hygiene product use

  - History of tampon, condom, diaphragm use

  - Postmenopausal

- **Sexual history:** risk factors for STDs, including unprotected intercourse and/or multiple partners

- **Medical history:** STDs

- **Social history:** drug, alcohol abuse

Focused Physical Exam
Genitourinary:

- Perform a complete pelvic exam in all cases.

- Closely evaluate external genitalia for lesions (vesicles, ulcers: syphilis or herpes; atrophy of vaginal walls: atrophic vaginitis).

- Perform speculum exam (strawberry cervix: trichomoniasis) and bimanual exam (cervical motion tenderness: cervicitis).

- Characterize vaginal discharge, including by pH and wet prep.

Evaluation and Management
See Table 23-6.

What to Tell the Patient

- For patients with STDs, be sure to reinforce safe sex practices and counsel patient to let partner(s) know so that the partner can be treated.

- For patients with yeast infections, over-the-counter antifungal preparations are equally effective as prescription vaginal creams.

- For patients with atrophic vaginitis, counsel patients that it may be a recurrent problem for postmenopausal women, especially if they are not on HRT.

TABLE 23-6.
EVALUATION AND MANAGEMENT OF PATIENTS WITH
VAGINAL DISCHARGE

Diagnosis	Physical findings and diagnostic tests	Treatment
Bacterial vaginosis (*Gardnerella vaginalis*)	Fishy-smelling, thin, homogeneous gray discharge. pH >4.5; KOH: (+) "whiff" test; wet prep: clue cells	Metronidazole, 500 mg PO bid ×7 days, MetroGel bid ×5 days, *or* clindamycin, 300 mg per vagina ×7 days
Candidiasis (*Candida albicans*)	White, curdy discharge; pruritus of vagina and labia. pH = 4.0–5.0; KOH: budding yeast, branching hyphae; recurrent infections: screen for diabetes	Fluconazole, 150 mg PO ×1 *or* Intravaginal: azole creams ×7–10 days Recurrent infections: fluconazole, 100 mg PO q wk, or clotrimazole vaginal suppository, 500 mg q wk ×6 mos
Trichomoniasis (*Trichomonas vaginalis*)	Profuse, watery, frothy, greenish discharge; "strawberry" cervix. pH = 5.0–6.0; wet prep: round, moving protozoa; motile flagella	Metronidazole, 2 g ×1 or 500 mg PO bid ×7 days *Treat sexual partner(s)*
Gonorrhea (*Neisseria gonorrhoeae*), chlamydia (*Chlamydia trachomatis*)	± Purulent discharge; ± friable cervix; may be asymptomatic. Gram stain and culture, DNA probe	Ceftriaxone, 125 mg IM ×1, or ciprofloxacin, 500 mg PO ×1 (for GC), *plus* azithromycin, 1 g PO ×1, or doxycycline, 100 mg PO bid ×7 days (for chlamydia) *Treat both infections* *Treat sexual partner(s)*
Atrophic vaginitis	Postmenopausal; vaginal dryness; dyspareunia; thin, atrophic vaginal walls. pH >4.5; wet prep: clumped epithelial cells	Estradiol vaginal cream, 1 g per vagina qd ×1–2 wks, then taper over 1–2 wks

(*continued*)

TABLE 23-6.
CONTINUED

Diagnosis	Physical findings and diagnostic tests	Treatment
Allergic vaginitis	Foul-smelling discharge; perineal irritation. pH <4.5; wet prep: WBCs	Discontinue use of product causing irritation
Foreign body	Foul-smelling or bloody discharge; vulvar erythema. Wet prep: WBCs	Remove foreign body

GC, gonococcal infection; KOH, potassium hydroxide.

SUGGESTED READING

American College of Obstetrics and Gynecology. *Management of anovulatory bleeding.* ACOG Practice Bulletin 14. Washington DC: ACOG, 2000.

Grady D, Herrington D, et al. Cardiovascular disease outcomes during 6.8 years of hormone therapy: Heart and Estrogen/Progestin Replacement Study Follow-up (HERS II). *JAMA* 2002;288(1):49–57.

Hatcher RA, Zieman M, Watt A, et al. *Managing contraception.* Tiger, GA: Bridging the Gap Foundation, 1999.

Hulley S, et al. Noncardiovascular disease outcomes during 6.8 years of hormone therapy: Heart and Estrogen/Progestin Replacement Study Follow-up (HERS II). *JAMA* 2002;288(1):58–66.

Hulley S, Grady D, et al. Randomized trial of estrogen plus progestin for secondary prevention of coronary heart disease on postmenopausal women. *JAMA* 1998;280:605–613.

Manson JE, Martin KA. Postmenopausal hormone-replacement therapy. *N Engl J Med* 2001;345(1):35–40.

Rossouw JE, Prentice RL, et al. Risks and benefits of estrogen plus progestin in healthy postmenopausal women: Principal results from the Women's Health Initiative Randomized Controlled Trial. *JAMA* 2002;288(3):321–333.

Shumaker SA, et al. Estrogen plus progestin and the incidence of dementia and mild cognitive impairment in postmenopausal women. The Women's Health Initative Memory Study: a randomized controlled trial. *JAMA* 2003;289:2651–2662.

Speroff L, Glass RH, Kase NG. *Clinical gynecologic endocrinology and infertility,* 6th ed. Philadelphia: Lippincott, Williams & Wilkins, 1999.

Stenchever MA, Droegemueller W, et al. *Comprehensive gynecology.* St. Louis: Mosby, 2001.

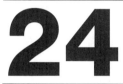

Miscellaneous Subjects

Everything but the kitchen sink . . .

PREOP EVALUATION

Preop management involves determining the risk for medical complications and maximizing a patient's medical condition before surgery. The majority of complications from surgery are cardiac, pulmonary, and infectious in etiology.

Key History

- **General:** type of surgery, medical condition leading to surgery, fever/chills (symptoms of infection), weight loss, obesity
- **Pulmonary:** shortness of breath, cough, dyspnea on exertion, sputum production
- **Cardiovascular:** chest pain, palpitations, orthopnea, paroxysmal nocturnal dyspnea
- **Extremities:** edema
- **Medical history:** heart disease (previous MI, arrhythmias, congestive heart failure), lung disease (COPD, asthma), diabetes, HTN, previous surgeries, previous complications from anesthesia
- **Family history:** reactions to anesthesia (malignant hyperthermia), delay in extubation
- **Social history:** tobacco/alcohol/drug use; anticipated needs at discharge (e.g., home health, rehabilitation facility, nursing home)
- **Medications:** comprehensive medication list (including over-the-counter medications, vitamins, and supplements)

Focused Physical Exam

- **Vital signs:** BP, heart rate, height/weight/BMI
- **General:** signs of malnutrition
- **HEENT:** carotid bruits, carotid upstroke, thyromegaly, jugular venous distention, temporal wasting
- **Pulmonary:** wheezes, rhonchi, prolonged expiratory phase, dullness to percussion
- **Cardiovascular:** rhythm, murmurs, gallops
- **Abdominal:** organomegaly

- **Extremities:** edema
- **Neurologic:** focal neurologic deficits

Evaluation

- **<40 yrs and healthy:** Consider CBC, urine hCG.
- **>40 yrs and healthy:** Consider CBC, ECG, blood glucose.
- **Cardiovascular disease:**
  - ECG, chest x-ray, CBC, electrolytes, BUN, creatinine, glucose.
- See cardiac risk assessment (Fig. 24-1).
- **Pulmonary disease:**
  - Good history anmd physical exam, chest x-ray, ECG, Hgb, electrolytes.
  - Consider pulmonary function tests (PFTs).
  - See Pulmonary Risk Assessment.
- **Malnutrition:** Serum albumin, CBC.
- See Table 24-1.

Pulmonary Risk Assessment

- **Risk factors for postop pulmonary complications:** smoking, poor general health, COPD, asthma, abdominal or thoracic surgery (the closer the surgery is to the diaphragm, the higher the risk), surgery >3 hrs' duration, general anesthesia, abnormal lung exam, unexplained cough or dyspnea, long-acting neuromuscular blockers (e.g., pancuronium).
- **Possible risk factors:**
  - P_{CO_2} >45 mm Hg on ABG, FEV_1/FVC <70%.
  - Obesity and age do not appear to be independent risk factors.
- **PFTs:**
  - Indicated for surgeries involving lung resection.
  - Consider ordering preop PFTs in the following patients:
    - Undergoing coronary artery bypass graft or upper abdominal surgery with a tobacco/dyspnea history
    - Undergoing lower abdominal surgery along with uncharacterized pulmonary disease
    - Undergoing any surgery with unexplained cough, dyspnea, or poor exercise tolerance
  - PFT results have not been demonstrated to predict postop pulmonary complications, so results not routinely used to exclude patient from surgery.

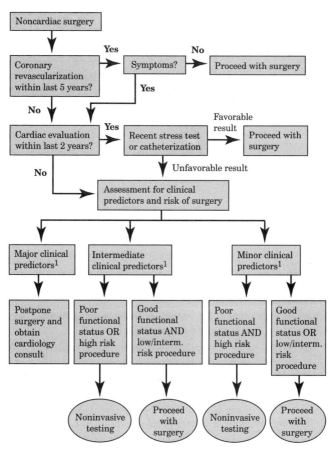

FIG. 24-1.
Cardiac risk stratification and testing. [1]See Table 24-1 for definitions of clinical predictors and of procedure risk. (From ACC/AHA guidelines for perioperative cardiovascular evaluation for noncardiac surgery. *Circulation* 1996;93:1280–1317.)

- **ABG:**

  - No absolute indication.

  - Some studies have shown that an elevated PCO_2 correlates with an increased risk of pulmonary complications. However, an elevated PCO_2 should not exclude a patient from surgery.

TABLE 24-1.
PROCEDURE RISK AND CLINICAL PREDICTORS

Procedure risk	Clinical predictors
High	**Major**
Emergency surgery	MI within past 6 wks
Anticipated major blood loss	Unstable angina
	Decompensated congestive heart failure
Vascular surgery (aortic/peripheral)	Significant arrhythmia
	Severe valvular disease
Intermediate	**Intermediate**
Abdominal or thoracic surgery	Mild angina
	Previous MI
Head or neck surgery	Compensated congestive heart failure
Carotid endarterectomy	Diabetes
Prostate surgery	Renal insufficiency
Orthopedic surgery	**Minor**
Low	Advanced age
Breast surgery	Abnormal ECG
Cataract surgery	Cardiac rhythm other than normal sinus rhythm
Superficial surgery	Low functional capacity (<4 mets[a])
Endoscopy	Previous stroke
	HTN

[a]mets = metabolic equivalents of O_2 consumption. >4 mets = good functional capacity (e.g., climbing one flight of stairs, jogging).

Malnutrition Assessment

- Malnutrition increases surgical morbidity and mortality.

- **Risk factors for malnutrition:** weight loss of >5% over 1 mo or >10% over 6 mos, serum albumin <3.2 mg/dL, total lymphocyte count of <3000.

- Consider preop supplements (Boost/Ensure, TPN) in severely malnourished patients.

PERIOP MANAGEMENT

- Consider periop beta blockers in high-risk cardiac patients; they have been shown to decrease periop cardiac morbidity and mortality.

  - Metoprolol, 25 mg PO bid.
  - Bisoprolol, 5–10 mg PO qd.

TABLE 24-2.
PERIOP MEDICATION CONSIDERATIONS

Medication	Suggested management
Aspirin, clopidogrel, *gingko biloba*, garlic supplements	Discontinue 1 wk before surgery to minimize risk of bleeding.
Beta blockers	Continue throughout periop period.
Calcium channel blockers	Continue throughout periop period.
Clonidine	Consider changing to clonidine patch before surgery until patient can take pills postop, as abrupt discontinuation may lead to severe rebound HTN.
Corticosteroids	For patients at risk for adrenal suppression (on chronic steroids or high dose for >3 wks), start stress-dose steroids the morning of surgery, usually hydrocortisone, 100 mg IV q6h.
Insulin	For type I diabetics: decrease insulin dose by $1/2$ on day of surgery.
	For type II diabetics: discontinue PO hypoglycemics the night before surgery and decrease insulin dose by $1/2$ on day of surgery.
NSAIDs	Discontinue >2 days before surgery.
Warfarin	If patient is at high risk for thromboembolism (recent DVT/PE, prosthetic valves):
	• Discontinue warfarin 2–3 days before surgery, then start heparin (unfractionated or LMWH) therapy from the time of discontinuation of warfarin until warfarin is restarted and therapeutic. Restart warfarin 1–2 days after surgery.
	• Hold LMWH dose the day of surgery, discontinue IV unfractionated heparin 2–3 hrs before surgery; resume postop.
	If patient has lower risk (distant CVA, AF):
	• Discontinue warfarin 2–3 days before surgery.
	• Resume 3–5 days after surgery.

AF, atrial fibrillation; CVA, cerebrovascular accident; DVT/PE, deep venous thrombosis/pulmonary embolism.

- Begin medication ≥1 wk preop; titrate to a heart rate of 60.
- Maximize pulmonary function with inhaled bronchodilators and inhaled corticosteroids.

- Consider a short course of oral corticosteroids periop if necessary.
- Consider antibiotics or delaying surgery if there are signs of infection.
- Evaluate for cause of unexplained cough or dyspnea.
- Advise patients to stop smoking 8 wks before surgery for maximum benefit.
- Recommend deep breathing exercises and incentive spirometry, particularly in patients with pulmonary disease and in patients undergoing thoracic or abdominal surgery.
- **Medication management:** See Table 24-2.

What to Tell the Patient

- Periop risks are primarily cardiac, pulmonary, and infectious in nature. All tests being ordered and medication adjustments made are designed to optimize the patient for surgery.
- Stop smoking.
- Deep breathing exercises and incentive spirometry can decrease postop pulmonary complications.

PAIN MANAGEMENT

- The key to managing chronic pain is to work with the patient to find the most effective modalities for pain control.
- Although addiction to narcotic pain medications is a concern, it is rare and should not prevent physicians from prescribing narcotics in appropriate situations.

Nonpharmacologic Therapies

- RICE (**r**est, **i**ce, **c**ompression, **e**levation) for acute musculoskeletal injuries
- Heat (after acute injury subsides)
- Physical therapy: an important adjunct to medications, particularly for chronic musculoskeletal pain

Pharmacotherapy

See WHO's guidelines for cancer pain management (Table 24-3), which are helpful for all types of pain.

Narcotics

- Equivalent doses for the narcotic analgesics can be found in Table 24-4.
- Be sure to prescribe a regular bowel regimen to minimize difficulties with constipation (e.g., senna, 1–2 tablets PO bid).
- Taper medications, especially opiates, to avoid withdrawal symptoms.

TABLE 24-3.
WHO GUIDELINES FOR CANCER PAIN MANAGEMENT

Intensity of pain	Treatment	Examples
Mild	24-hr coverage with nonopioid ± adjuvant[a]	Aspirin, 650 mg PO q4–6h
		Acetaminophen, 650 mg PO q4–6h
		Ibuprofen, 200–800 mg PO q6–8h
Mild to moderate	Weak opioid + nonopioid agent ± adjuvant[a]	Acetaminophen + codeine (Tylenol #3), 1–2 tablets PO q4–6h
		Hydrocodone (Vicodin), 1–2 tablets PO q4–6h
		Oxycodone (Percocet/Percodan), 1–2 tabs PO q4–6h
Moderate to severe	Strong opioid ± nonopioid ± adjuvant[a]	Morphine IR, 30 mg PO q4h
		Morphine sulfate (MS Contin), 30 mg PO q8–12h
		Oxycodone (OxyContin), 10–40 mg PO q12h
		Fentanyl patch, 25–100 μg q72h

[a]Adjuvant medications include agents that (1) decrease neuropathic pain (anticonvulsants [e.g., carbamazepine], antidepressants [especially tricyclic antidepressants]), (2) relieve itching (antihistamines [hydroxyzine]), (3) relieve anxiety (benzodiazepines), and (4) relieve muscle spasms (muscle relaxants [e.g., cyclobenzaprine], benzodiazepines).
From World Health Organization. *Cancer pain relief and palliative care: report of a WHO expert committee, technical report series.* 1990:804, with permission.

TABLE 24-4.
EQUIVALENT DOSES FOR NARCOTIC ANALGESICS

Drug	Dose for equivalent analgesia
Strong opioids:	
Morphine	30 mg (short acting); 90 mg (long acting)
Hydromorphone	7.5 mg
Fentanyl	25–50 μg
Weak opioids:	
Codeine	30–60 mg
Oxycodone	5–10 mg
Hydrocodone	5–10 mg

TABLE 24-5.
MEDICATIONS FOR NEUROPATHIC PAIN

Class	Examples
Tricyclic antidepressants	Amitriptyline, 25–100 mg PO qhs
	Nortriptyline, 10–150 mg PO qhs
	Desipramine, 10–300 mg PO qhs
Anticonvulsants	Carbamazepine, 200 mg PO bid
	Clonazepam, 0.5 mg PO qd
GABA inhibitor	Gabapentin, 300–600 mg PO bid–tid
Substance P inhibitor	Capsaicin cream, 0.025% topical tid

Medications for Neuropathic Pain

- See Table 24-5.

- Start at a low dose and increase as tolerated.

- Tricyclic antidepressants are very sedating (good for patients with concurrent sleep difficulties or depression). Avoid in suicidal patients (potentially fatal in overdose situation).

- Monitor CBC in patients taking carbamazepine (myelosuppression).

Difficult Management Situations

- **Patients abusing medications ("drug seekers"):**

  - Set firm boundaries and stick to them.

  - Establish a contract with the patient detailing a specific plan. Make clear to patient that if the agreement is broken, you will no longer provide care to them. Alert all members of the care team of the contract terms.

  - Document in the chart (contract details, amount/when medication prescribed).

- Some patients may give you **disability forms** to fill out. Honesty is the best policy for these forms (you may disagree with your patient's "self-assessment").

- **Somatization disorder:** Consistent medical care and frequent visits can prevent overmedication and/or unnecessary medication.

- **Do not undertreat pain for fear of causing patient addiction.** It is rare for a patient without a history of substance abuse and in legitimate pain to become a medication addict (<1%).

TABLE 24-6.
COMMON ANALGESIC SIDE EFFECTS

Drug class	Major side effects
Aspirin	Increased risk of GI bleeding
	Increased bruising, bleeding
	Avoid in patients <18 (Reye's syndrome)
Acetaminophen	Taking >4 g/day or taking with alcohol increases risk of hepatotoxicity
NSAIDs	Increased GI bleeding (lower with COX-2 inhibitors)
	Acute renal failure/interstitial nephritis
	GI effects (dyspepsia, nausea, abdominal pain)
Muscle relaxants	Drowsiness (avoid operating heavy machinery, etc.)
	Dry mouth
	Dizziness, blurred vision
	GI effects (nausea, dyspepsia)
Narcotics	Dizziness
	Sedation (avoid operating heavy machinery, etc.)
	GI effects (nausea, vomiting, constipation)
	Urinary retention
	Pruritus
	Respiratory depression
Tramadol (Ultram)	Dizziness
	GI effects (nausea, constipation, diarrhea)
	Somnolence

When to Refer

- Consider referring the patient to a specialized pain clinic if you cannot achieve adequate pain control.
- Consider a referral to a psychiatrist for patients with somatization disorder.

What to Tell the Patient

- Chronic pain is a difficult problem, and it may take several modes of treatment to get the pain under control.
- Addiction to prescribed narcotics is rare. Tolerance to the medication, which results in a need for increased dose to achieve analgesia, is common but is *not* the same as dependence.

- All pain medications have potentially serious side effects (Table 24-6).

PERIPHERAL ARTERIAL DISEASE

Peripheral arterial disease (PAD) is caused by atherosclerotic occlusion of the arteries to the legs.

Risk Factors

- **Older age**

- **Smoking:** 2–5× increased risk (>80% patients with claudication are former or current smokers)

- **Diabetes:** 3–4× increased risk; extensive, severe PAD with calcification

- **Hypercholesterolemia**

- **HTN:** 2.5× increased risk in men, 4× increased risk in women (Framingham Heart Study)

- **Hyperhomocystinemia:** 2–3× increased risk

Key History

- **Symptoms of claudication** (33% of patients with PAD):

  - Pain in one or both calves (thigh and/or buttock).

  - Discomfort does not go away with continued walking but is relieved with rest.

  - Critical leg ischemia (5% of patients with PAD): ischemic pain at rest relieved with dangling leg over edge of bed, ulceration, gangrene.

- **Social history:** tobacco use

- **Medical history:** HTN, hyperlipidemia, coronary artery disease, diabetes, atrial fibrillation, cerebrovascular disease

Focused Physical Exam

- **Vascular:** carotid, abdominal, femoral bruits, diminished peripheral pulses (compare vs contralateral side)

- **Extremities:** atrophic changes in the skin; SC tissue atrophy; muscle weakness/atrophy; pallor; paresthesias; paralysis; dependent rubor; cool skin; ulceration/fissures; gangrene; loose, brittle toenails

Evaluation

Ankle/Brachial Indices (ABIs)

- Ratio of SBP measured at ankle to SBP in brachial artery.

TABLE 24-7.
CLASSIFICATION OF PERIPHERAL ARTERIAL DISEASE (PAD) BASED ON ANKLE/BRACHIAL INDEX

Classification	Ankle/brachial index
Normal	>1
Mild to moderate PAD (usually symptomatic)	0.9–0.41
Severe PAD (may have critical limb ischemia)	0.41–0

From Hiatt WR. Medical treatment of peripheral arterial disease and claudication. *N Engl J Med* 2001;344(21):1608–1621, with permission.

- Can be performed in the office with Doppler probe.
- ABI <0.9 is considered abnormal (95% sensitive for angiographically significant PAD).
- The lower the ABI, the higher the risk for death from a cardiovascular event (Table 24-7).

Duplex U/S

Noninvasive assessment of peripheral artery anatomy and functional significance of stenoses as related to flow

Treadmill Exercise Testing

- "Extremity stress test": allows clinical correlation between arterial stenoses and exercise capacity and development of symptoms.
- Patients with PAD often also have coronary artery disease, so consider performing cardiac stress testing as well.

Contrast Angiography

Indicated for evaluation of arterial anatomy before revascularization surgery.

Magnetic Resonance Angiography

Substitution for conventional angiography in patients at risk for contrast-related complications (renal failure, iodine allergy).

Management
Goals

- Decrease claudication/resting limb pain.
- Preserve limb function/viability.
- Decrease concomitant cardiovascular risk (MI, stroke, death).

Conservative Measures

- Daily walking programs for fixed periods of time. Goal should be to walk ≥20 mins 3×/day (increase time as tolerated).

- Secondary prevention is risk factor modification:

  - Control HTN: goal BP <130/85 (see Chap. 8, Cardiology). Caution with beta blockers, as they may worsen claudication.

  - Control lipids: goal for low-density lipoprotein with CAD: <100 (see Chap. 8, Cardiology).

  - Tobacco cessation (50% decreased mortality at 5 yrs).

  - Check homocysteine level: if increased, folic acid, 1 mg PO qd.

  - Control diabetes (see Chap. 10, Endocrinology).

- **Drug therapy:**

  - **Pentoxifylline (Trental),** 400 mg PO tid with meals. Has small effects on walking distance (20% increase in distance before development of absolute claudication).

  - **Cilostazol (Pletal),** 100 mg PO bid on empty stomach.

    - Results in increased pain-free and maximal treadmill walking distance, increased ABIs, and increased HDL levels.

    - Coadministration with ASA is considered safe; decrease dose with azoles, erythromycin, diltiazem, omeprazole.

    - Contraindicated in patients with heart failure.

    - Side effect: headache.

  - **Antiplatelet drug therapy** (indicated in all patients with PAD):

    - **ASA,** 81–325 mg PO qd.

    - **Clopidogrel (Plavix),** 75 mg PO qd in ASA-intolerant patients.

When to Refer

Consider surgical or angioplastic treatment for patients who can tolerate surgery and in whom PAD significantly interferes with activities of daily living.

Difficult Management Situations

- Diabetics (especially those who smoke): increased risk for PAD at an early age.

  - Ulcers that result from PAD are often slow to heal and become infected.

- Diabetic neuropathy increases risk of ulceration.

- Poor vision may limit proper foot care.

- Regular appointments to diabetic foot clinic may decrease limb loss by ≥50%.

What to Tell the Patient

- Risk factor modification is key to decreasing risk of limb loss (especially tobacco cessation).

- Exercise program participation will decrease pain and improve quality of life.

- Extremity stenosis/pain is a harbinger for other vascular blockages and ischemia and warrants a thorough cardiovascular evaluation.

- Vascular surgery is a high-risk procedure: the risks and benefits must be individually weighed.

UNINTENTIONAL WEIGHT LOSS

After age 60, there is a gradual decline in weight, particularly in muscle mass. Excessive weight loss is associated with increased morbidity and mortality.

Differential Diagnosis and Key History

See Table 24-8.

Focused Physical Exam

- **Vital signs:** weight (compare with old record)

- **HEENT:** temporal wasting, dry mouth, poor vision

- **Cardiovascular:** tachycardia, irregular rhythm (atrial fibrillation/ hyperthyroidism)

- **Abdominal:** tenderness, masses (malignancy)

- **Rectal:** prostate mass, rectal mass, heme-positive stools (malignancy)

- **Lymph:** complete lymph node exam (malignancy)

- **Breast and pelvic:** masses (malignancy)

- **Neurologic:** tremor, focal deficits

- **Psychiatric:** Mini-Mental Status Exam (see Chap. 12, Geriatrics), depression/anxiety assessment

Evaluation

- In approximately 90% of cases, a diagnosis can be made based on history and physical exam.

TABLE 24-8.
DIFFERENTIAL DIAGNOSIS AND KEY HISTORY IN UNINTENTIONAL WEIGHT LOSS

Symptom/sign	Key history
Anorexia	Neuropsychiatric illness (depression/dementia)
	Medical illness (CHF, PUD, COPD, uremia)
	Medications
	Restricted diets
	Anorexia nervosa
Difficulty eating	Dysphagia/odynophagia
	Poorly fitting dentures
	Anticholinergic medications that cause dry mouth
	Visual impairment
	Tremor
Weight loss despite normal caloric intake	Endocrine: diabetes, thyroid disease
	GI disease: chronic pancreatitis, sprue
	Occult malignancy (GI, pancreas, liver, leukemia, lymphoma, lung, breast)
	Infection (HIV, TB, hepatitis)
	AIDS wasting syndrome
	Bulimia
Social/socioeconomic problems	Loss of spouse
	Reliance on others to shop for food/cook
	Inability to feed one's self
	Low income

CHF, congestive heart failure; PUD, peptic ulcer disease.

- Lab evaluation: CBC, Chem 12, UA, TSH, fecal occult blood testing, chest x-ray, Pap smear, and mammogram at a minimum.
- Consider UGI or EGD, as esophagitis/peptic ulcer disease may be silent.
- Consider colonoscopy (especially if >50).
- Refer to a dietitian for a more complete dietary assessment (e.g., calorie counts).
- CT scan (chest/abdominal/pelvis scan) or additional lab tests should be based on the history and physical exam.

Management

Management is based on the diagnosis.

- Treat medical illnesses (diabetes, thyroid disease, congestive heart failure, COPD, infection, peptic ulcer disease, esophagitis, cirrhosis, inflammatory bowel disease, chronic pancreatitis, sprue).

- Treat psychiatric illness. Refer patients with anorexia nervosa or bulimia to a psychiatrist and dietitian for more specialized care.

- Withdraw all unnecessary medications.

- Consider nutritional supplements (e.g., Boost or Ensure, 1 can tid between meals).

- For certain situations, consider an appetite stimulant (mirtazapine [Remeron], 15 mg PO qhs; megestrol [Megace] suspension, 400 mg PO bid for AIDS wasting syndrome; or cyproheptadine [Periactin], 8 mg PO qid for anorexia nervosa).

- For patients with difficulty shopping or cooking, refer to a social worker or the state's Department of Aging for assistance (e.g., Meals on Wheels).

- Provide vitamin supplementation with a multivitamin, 1 tablet PO qd.

When to Refer

- Consider referring those patients in need of endoscopy, those with end-stage liver disease, and inflammatory bowel disease to a gastroenterologist/hepatologist.

- Refer those with cancer to an oncologist.

- Refer those with financial needs to a social worker or the Department of Aging to help arrange for Meals on Wheels, appliances to help with feeding, or a chore worker for shopping, cooking, and feeding.

- Refer those who have functional limitations/dysphagia secondary to past cerebrovascular accidents or chronic deconditioning to a physical therapist, occupational therapist, and speech therapist.

- Have all patients evaluated by a nutritionist to assess caloric needs.

What to Tell the Patient

- Weight loss is common as people age, but sustained/rapid weight loss often has an underlying cause.

- Weight loss carries with it morbidity and mortality from the weight loss itself but also from the underlying cause.

WEAKNESS

Definition

- Weakness is a vague complaint that patients may use to describe fatigue, malaise, dizziness, or even shortness of breath.

- A thorough history and review of systems is key to further define the problem.

Differential Diagnosis

- **Autoimmune:** dermatomyositis/polymyositis, SLE, rheumatoid arthritis

- **Cardiovascular:** orthostasis, arrhythmia, coronary artery disease, valvular disease, congestive heart failure

- **Endocrine:** diabetes, hypothyroidism

- **Hematologic:** anemia, leukemia, lymphoma, myeloma

- **Iatrogenic:** overmedication, polypharmacy

- **Infectious:** upper respiratory infection, pneumonia, TB, UTI, HIV, viral hepatitis

- **Malignancy:** lung, colon, breast, cervical, prostate

- **Metabolic:** hypokalemia, renal failure (acute or chronic), volume depletion

- **Neurologic:** cerebrovascular accident, myasthenia gravis, amyotrophic lateral sclerosis, myopathy, Guillain-Barré syndrome, MS

- **Pulmonary:** COPD, obstructive sleep apnea

- **Psychiatric:** depression, drug use, alcoholism

- **Other:** fibromyalgia, chronic fatigue syndrome

Key History and Physical Exam

See Table 24-9.

Evaluation

- **Screening labs:** CBC, electrolytes, LFTs, TSH, ESR, creatine kinase, aldolase

- **ECG**

- **Other tests to consider:**
  - **UA** for infection
  - **Chest x-ray** to rule out lung disease, malignancy
  - **Cardiac evaluation:** echocardiogram

TABLE 24-9.
PHYSICAL EXAM AND KEY HISTORY IN
PATIENTS WITH WEAKNESS

Symptoms/signs	Suggested diagnosis
Blurred or double vision, muscle weakness, dysphagia	Neurologic disorders (myasthenia gravis, MS)
Daytime somnolence, snoring	Obstructive sleep apnea
Diuretics, beta blockers, benzodiazepines, opioids, antipsychotics, antidepressants, anticonvulsants, antihistamines, oral hypoglycemics	Medication side effects
Dysarthria, focal neurologic deficit	Cerebrovascular disease
Dyspnea, cough, leg swelling, wheezing	Congestive heart failure, anemia, COPD
Easy bruising, fatigue, weight loss	Leukemia
Fever/chills, night sweats	Infection, malignancy
High-risk sexual behavior, substance abuse	HIV, hepatitis
Insomnia, anhedonia, depressed mood	Depression
Lymphadenopathy	Lymphoma
Menorrhagia	Anemia
Rash, joint pain/swelling, fatigue	Dermatomyositis, SLE, rheumatoid arthritis
Tenderness at "trigger points"	Fibromyalgia
Weight gain, cold intolerance, fatigue	Hypothyroidism
Weight loss, guaiac-positive stool	Malignancy

- **CT scan or MRI of brain/spinal cord:** if suspected cerebrovascular accident or other neurologic disorder (e.g., radiculopathy, MS, spinal cord compression)
- **Infection workup:** PPD, HIV, acute hepatitis panel
- **Malignancy screening:** mammogram, Pap smear, prostate screening antigen, flexible sigmoidoscopy or colonoscopy
- **ANA, serum protein electrophoresis/urine protein electrophoresis** if the history suggests rheumatologic disease or malignancy
- **Electromyography or nerve conduction study** for muscle weakness or suspected neuropathy

Management

- Treat any underlying conditions.

- Closely evaluate the patient's list of medications, including any over-the-counter drugs; discontinue any offending medications.

Red Flags

- Patients with objective neurologic deficits need further workup.

- Hospitalize patients with acute stroke.

When to Refer

Consider referral to neurologist if patient has true muscle weakness/neurologic deficits.

What to Tell the Patient

If all findings are normal, provide reassurance.

COMPLEMENTARY AND ALTERNATIVE MEDICINE

Alternative therapies can range from entire systems to use of a single herbal supplement. This section details a few of the major alternative systems as well as some of the commonly used supplements (Tables 24-10 and 24-11).

Acupuncture

- Traditional practice of East Asia that is sometimes used in conjunction with herbal therapies.

- Used to treat a variety of conditions, from chronic pain to chronic illnesses.

- Needles are inserted into defined sites to regulate and balance *chi*, a kind of energy that promotes health.

- There is good evidence that acupuncture is effective for postop pain and chemotherapy-induced nausea and vomiting. May also be effective for chronic pain syndromes, migraine headaches, and menstrual cramps.

- Risks include trauma to the spine, pneumothorax, and infection (from unsterilized needles).

Chiropractic Therapy

- Used to treat musculoskeletal disorders via manipulation of the spine.

- Likely effective short-term therapy for low back pain and neck pain, although long-term efficacy remains to be proven. May also be effective for headache.

- Risks include trauma to the spine (particularly when cervical spine is manipulated), vertebral fracture, disk herniation, and, rarely, cauda equina syndrome.

Homeopathy

- Uses substances that produce certain symptoms in healthy individuals to treat identical symptoms in sick people.

- The substances used are extremely diluted, at times to the point that the original substance may not remain in the dilution at all.

- Few studies have been done regarding efficacy.

- Homeopathic preparations can have additives that are potentially toxic, such as cadmium and arsenic.

Naturopathy

- Encompasses a wide assortment of therapies, including herbal therapy, use of dietary supplements, homeopathy, counseling, and manipulation. It can include massage therapy that is used to treat conditions other than musculoskeletal conditions.

- Few studies have been done regarding efficacy.

- Risks depend on the treatments being given.

Osteopathy

- Once similar to chiropractic medicine, osteopathic physicians (D.O.s) are now the equivalent of allopathic physicians (M.D.s).

- Some patients who see osteopathic physicians still receive manipulative therapy and incur risks similar to those incurred by patients who see chiropractors.

What to Tell the Patient

- Complementary and alternative therapies can be useful for treatment of certain disorders. However, "natural" or "supplement" does not always mean safe. **All treatments have potential side effects** that may be unpleasant or even dangerous.

- **Herbal and dietary supplements are not regulated by the FDA.** Therefore, the concentration and purity of such supplements are not guaranteed, and they may contain harmful substances.

- **Supplements are medications:** Stick to the recommended dosage and be aware of side effects and medication interactions.

- Be sure to tell the physician **every pill** you are taking, including over-the-counter medications, vitamins, herbal supplements, and dietary supplements.

TABLE 24-10.
COMMON HERBAL MEDICINES

Herb	Common uses	Notes
Black cohosh (*Cimicifuga racemosa*)	Dysmenor-rhea Menopausal symptoms	*Mechanism*: binds to estrogen receptors, decreases LH secretion. *Evidence*: studies show efficacy at 8 mg/day. *Dosage*: 8 mg PO qd. *Side effects*: gastric discomfort, dizziness, nausea. *Safety*: caution with anticoagulants; may cause bleeding; may potentiate antihypertensive medications. *Contraindications*: oral contraceptives, estrogen.
Echinacea (*E. angustifolia, E. pallida, E. purpurea*)	Treatment of URI Tincture used for wound healing	*Mechanism*: stimulates both humoral and cellular immunity. *Evidence*: studies regarding efficacy had mixed results. Echinacea likely not very effective for prevention of URI, but may be effective for treatment. *Dosage*: take 300–400 mg PO tid of dried extract at onset of symptoms for 7–10 days. *E. purpurea* tincture: apply topically to healing wound. *Side effects*: mild GI upset; can exacerbate atopic conditions or autoimmune disease. *Safety*: generally regarded as safe. *Contraindications*: patients allergic to the daisy family (anaphylaxis reported).
Feverfew (*Tanacetum parthenium*)	Migraine prophylaxis	*Mechanism*: causes vasodilation and reduces inflammation; may also inhibit platelet aggregation. *Evidence*: randomized double-blinded placebo-controlled trial demonstrated 70% reduction in migraine frequency and severity. *Dosage*: 25–75 mg PO bid of 0.2% parthenolide extract.

(continued)

TABLE 24-10.
CONTINUED

Herb	Common uses	Notes
		Side effects: aphthous ulcers, GI irritation, rebound headaches.
		Safety: no long-term safety data. May potentiate antiplatelet medications.
		Contraindications: pregnancy.
Garlic (*Allium sativum*)	Decreases cholesterol Lowers BP	*Mechanism*: active ingredient is allicin, which inhibits hepatic cholesterol synthesis.
		Evidence: trials show decrease in LDL of 10–13.5 mg/dL and decrease in triglycerides of 7–30 mg/dL at 3 mos; however, long-term trial showed no difference in rate of MI at 3 yrs. Some trials also found 5–7% decrease in BP.
		Dosage: 1 fresh clove PO qd or 300 mg PO bid–tid.
		Side effects: halitosis, body odor, abdominal pain.
		Safety: generally regarded as safe.
		Contraindications: none.
		Drug interactions: decreases serum levels of saquinavir; may increase INR with warfarin.
Ginkgo (*Ginkgo biloba*)	Alzheimer's disease Multiinfarct dementia Claudication	*Mechanism*: inhibits platelet activating factor; also has vasoregulatory and antioxidant effects.
		Evidence: studies demonstrate delay in decline of cognitive function in patients with mild to moderate dementia; increases pain-free walking distance by 50% in patients with claudication.
		Dosage: 40 mg PO tid or 80 mg PO bid.
		Side effects: Mild GI upset, headache, dizziness.
		Safety: serious adverse effects include intracranial bleeding, seizures.
		Contraindications: advise patients to stop supplements >1 wk before surgical procedures to decrease risk of bleeding.

(continued)

TABLE 24-10.
CONTINUED

Herb	Common uses	Notes
Ginseng (*Panax ginseng*)	Increases well-being, decreases fatigue / Aphrodisiac	*Mechanism*: stimulation of CNS, modulation of T cells, acceleration of hepatic lipogenesis. *Evidence*: no evidence supporting use for increasing energy levels or well-being. *Dosage*: 0.5–2 g root or 200–600 mg extract PO qd. *Side effects*: insomnia, diarrhea, vaginal bleeding, headache, HTN, hypotension. *Safety*: Stevens-Johnson syndrome has been reported. *Contraindications*: patients with coronary artery disease, HTN, diabetes. *Drug interactions*: may be potentiated by stimulants; do not use with MAOIs, hypoglycemic agents, warfarin.
Kava (*Piper methysticum*)	Anxiety / Insomnia	*Mechanism*: kavapyrones have anxiolytic, analgesic, muscle relaxant properties. May act at GABA receptors. *Evidence*: randomized, placebo-controlled trials demonstrate that kava is better than placebo in relieving anxiety. *Dosage*: 60–100 mg PO tid. *Side effects*: allergic skin reaction, GI upset. In high doses, kava can cause a reversible ichthyosiform eruption accompanied by eye irritation (kava dermopathy). *Safety*: linked to cases of hepatitis, cirrhosis, and liver failure. *Contraindications*: severe depression. *Drug interactions*: may potentiate effects of alcohol, antidepressants, benzodiazepines.
Ma huang (*Ephedra sinica*)	Asthma	*Mechanism*: vasodilator, circulatory stimulant, bronchodilator. Contains ephedrine and pseudoephedrine.

(*continued*)

TABLE 24-10.
CONTINUED

Herb	Common uses	Notes
	Decongestant Obesity Stimulant	*Evidence*: ma huang is effective as decongestant and bronchodilator. Combined with caffeine, also effective for weight loss.
		Dosage: limit to 8 mg PO/dose or 24 mg PO qd.
		Side effects: dry mouth, insomnia, palpitations, anxiety, increased BP.
		Safety: has been linked to strokes, MI, seizures, and death.
		Contraindications: patients with coronary artery disease, stroke, seizure history. Do not use in patients taking beta blockers, MAOIs, phenothiazines, theophylline.
Saw palmetto (*Serenoa repens*)	Benign prostatic hyperplasia	*Mechanism*: inhibits 5-alpha-reductase and inhibits dihydrotestosterone binding to cytosolic androgen receptors.
		Evidence: randomized controlled trials demonstrate equal efficacy to finasteride in decreasing nocturia and increasing urinary flow.
		Dosage: 160 mg PO bid of lipophilic extract.
		Side effects: mild GI upset, headache, mild diuretic effects.
		Safety: generally safe.
St. John's wort (*Hypericum perforatum*)	Depression	*Mechanism*: inhibits dopamine, norepinephrine, and serotonin in high doses. Causes MAO inhibition *in vitro*.
		Evidence: randomized, placebo-controlled trials show efficacy for mild to moderate depression. Efficacy is similar to low-dose tricyclic antidepressants and SSRIs.
		Dosage: 300 mg PO tid; can titrate up to 1000 mg qd.
		Side effects: nausea, fatigue, restlessness, photosensitization.
		Safety: serious side effects rare; can induce mania.

(*continued*)

**TABLE 24-10.
CONTINUED**

Herb	Common uses	Notes
		Contraindications: do not combine with other antidepressants (can cause serotonin syndrome).
		Drug interactions: induces cytochrome p450 system.
Valerian (*Valeriana officinalis*)	Sedative	*Mechanism*: unknown.
		Evidence: randomized double-blind, placebo-controlled trial demonstrated improved sleep quality with no hangover effects noted.
		Dosage: 400–900 mg PO qhs, take 30 mins before bedtime.
		Side effects: headaches, restlessness, palpitations. No abuse potential.
		Contraindications: pregnancy.
		Drug interactions: may potentiate effects of other sedatives.
Yohimbine (*Pausinystalia yohimbe*)	Impotence	*Mechanism*: alpha blocker, causes vasodilation.
		Evidence: limited efficacy, mainly in patients with psychogenic erectile dysfunction.
		Dosage: 5.4 mg PO tid.
		Side effects: stomach discomfort, fatigue, weakness, increased BP, anxiety, palpitations, headache, urinary frequency.
		Safety: overdose can cause weakness, paralysis, and death.
		Contraindications: caution in patients with cardiac disease, liver disease, renal disease, diabetes.
		Drug interactions: MAOIs, phenylpropanolamine.

TABLE 24-11.
COMMON VITAMINS AND SUPPLEMENTS

Name	Common uses	Notes
Arginine	Claudication	Endothelial vasodilator, improves blood flow.
		Dosage: 8–21 g qd.
		Generally safe.
Glucosamine/ chondroitin	Osteoarthritis	Studies show 1500 mg/day of glucosamine and chondroitin to have beneficial effects in OA.
		Generally safe.
Melatonin	Jet lag	Can cause depression.
	Sleep disorders	
Pantothenic acid (niacin)	Hyperlipidemia	Decreases low-density lipoprotein; increases high-density lipoprotein.
		High doses (>1000 mg qd) should be used only under physician supervision.
		Side effects: flushing (can decrease by taking aspirin 30 mins before niacin), diarrhea, rare hepatitis.
Soy	Menopause	Ingestion of 20 g/day has been shown to decrease hot flashes; 30–40 g/day has been shown to decrease cholesterol. Also increases bone density.
	Decreases cholesterol	
		Safe.
Vitamin A	Used to treat psoriasis, acne, and epithelial cell cancers	Teratogenic.
		Side effects: headaches, bone pain, dermatitis, and at high doses, liver toxicity.
Vitamin B_2	Migraine prophylaxis	No clear evidence of efficacy. Generally safe.
Vitamin B_6	Carpal tunnel syndrome	High doses can cause sensory neuropathy.
	PMS	
	Nausea/vomiting of pregnancy	

(continued)

TABLE 24-11.
CONTINUED

Name	Common uses	Notes
Vitamin C	Colds	Safe up to 1 g qd.
		Side effects: diarrhea, kidney stones at high doses. Can increase iron absorption.
Vitamin D	Osteoporosis	Side effects: weakness, fatigue, head-ache, vomiting, hypercalcemia/hyper-calciuria, and renal dysfunction at high doses.
	Renal osteodystro-phy	
	Psoriasis	Deficiency is rare.
Vitamin E	Alzheimer's dis-ease	Antioxidant activity.
		Studies have shown that 2000 IU/day for Alzheimer's patients delays place-ment into nursing home by 4–6 mos.
		Recent studies have not shown benefit for prevention of heart disease.

SUGGESTED READING

ACC/AHA Guidelines for perioperative cardiovascular evaluation for non-cardiac surgery. *Circulation* 1996;93:1280–1317.

Blumenthal M, Gruenwald J, et al. German commission e monographs: medicinal plants for human use. Austin, TX: American Botanical Council, 1998.

Fontanarosa PB, ed. *Alternative medicine: an objective assessment*. Chicago: American Medical Association, 2000.

Gazewood JD, Mehr DR. Diagnosis and management of weight loss in the elderly. *J Fam Pract* 1999;47:19–25.

Goldman L, et al. Multifactoral index of cardiac risk in noncardiac surgical procedures. *N Engl J Med* 1977;297:845–850.

Hiatt WR. Medical treatment of peripheral arterial disease and claudication. *N Engl J Med* 2001:344(21)1608–1621.

Levy MH. Pharmacologic treatment of cancer pain. *N Engl J Med* 1996; 335:1124–1132.

McDermott MM, et al. Leg symptoms, the ankle-brachial index, and walking ability in patients with peripheral vascular disease. *J Gen Intern Med* 1999;14:173–181.

National Center for Complementary and Alternative Medicine (NIH). www.nccam.nih.gov. Last accessed: May 19, 2003.

Nehler MR, Hiatt WR. Exercise therapy for claudication. *Ann Vasc Surg* 1999;13:109–114.

Smetana GW. Preoperative pulmonary evaluation. *N Engl J Med* 1999; 340(12):937–944.

Tyler VE. *Herbs of choice: the therapeutic use of phytomedicinals.* Binghamton, NY: Pharmaceutical Products Press, 1994.

World Health Organization. Cancer pain relief and palliative care: Report of a WHO expert committee, technical report series. 804. 1990.

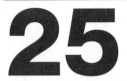 # Procedures

A chance to cut is a chance to cure . . .

DERMATOLOGY PROCEDURES
Potassium Hydroxide (KOH) Prep

- **Indications:** diagnosis of fungal infections

- **Contraindications:** none

- **What you will need:** 10% or 20% KOH, no. 15 scalpel, microscopic slide, cover slip, paper towel, microscope, alcohol lamp or plate warmer (optional)

- **Procedure:**

  1. Using scalpel blade, vigorously scrape scale from a lesion onto a microscopic slide. Avoid scraping very thick pieces of scale, as they are more difficult to examine.
  2. Place 2 drops of KOH solution directly on the slide.
  3. Cover slide with a cover slip.
  4. Allow slide to dry slightly. By use of an alcohol lamp or plate warmer, gently heat the slide until the bottom of the slide is warm. Avoid boiling the sample.
  5. Blot off excess KOH by placing slide in a paper towel and applying firm pressure to top and bottom of slide. This also spreads the cells into a thick layer on the slide for better visualization under the microscope.
  6. Examine slide under the microscope, using low illumination for easier identification of hyphae.
  7. Scan the entire slide under low power (10×). Use the high dry power objective (45×) for positive confirmation of hyphae.

Cryosurgery (Liquid Nitrogen/LN₂)

- **Indications:** removal of warts, actinic keratosis, skin tags

- **Contraindications:** none

- **What you will need:** liquid nitrogen in a proper dispenser

- **Procedure:**

  1. No skin preparation or local anesthetic is required.
  2. Instruct patient that liquid nitrogen will initially feel cold, then burn. Steady lesion as much as possible. Caution near eyes or mucous membranes.

3. Apply liquid nitrogen to lesion using a cotton-dipped swab or direct spray. When using direct spray, a pulsatile motion covering the lesion only as much as necessary is preferred. Spray the lesion for 7–15 secs.

4. Application may be repeated once after allowing the lesion to thaw.

5. Subsequent burning and swelling with blister formation usually occur. Pay particular attention to body site and skin thickness.

Shave Biopsy

• **Indications:** Evaluation of skin lesion or rash.

• **Contraindications: If there is any suspicion of melanoma, do not perform a shave biopsy!**

• **What you will need:** Betadine, 1% lidocaine, scalpel blade, sterile forceps, gauze, specimen cup filled with formalin, sterile gloves.

• **Procedure:**

1. Clean and sterilize biopsy site and adjacent area with Betadine. Pay particular attention to location of the biopsy (marking the lesion with an ink pen may be done), as the lesion may be more difficult to identify after Betadine application.

2. Local anesthesia is administered using 1% lidocaine. Using the anesthetic injection, make a wheal over the lesion.

3. Shave area with a scalpel blade using a slight scooping motion. Remember, a biopsy is done to sample a lesion, not necessarily to excise the lesion.

4. Using forceps, remove sample and place in a specimen cup filled with formalin solution.

5. Hemostasis is achieved at site with gauze application and proper pressure.

6. A dressing may be applied at the site.

Punch Biopsy

• **Indications:** to evaluate a skin lesion

• **Contraindications:** none

• **What you will need:** Betadine, 1% lidocaine, punch biopsy instrument (common sizes are 3, 4, and 6 mm), sterile forceps, sterile scissors, suture, gauze, specimen cup filled with formalin, sterile gloves

• **Procedure:**

1. Clean and sterilize biopsy site and adjacent area with Betadine. Pay particular attention to the location of the biopsy (marking the lesion with an ink pen may be done), as the lesion may be more difficult to identify after Betadine application.

2. Local anesthesia is administered using 1% lidocaine. Using anesthetic injection, make a wheal over the lesion.

3. Insert punch biopsy instrument over the biopsy site. Gently lift the punch biopsy after skin penetration is achieved (biopsy sample will usually lift up with the instrument).

4. Using forceps, gently lift the sample enough to snip it off at the SC fat level. Place sample in a specimen cup filled with formalin solution. Be particularly careful to avoid damaging tissue with the forceps.

5. Place the appropriate amount of sutures to close the skin defect and achieve hemostasis.

6. Apply dressing to the sutured site and provide proper wound care instructions.

7. Remove sutures in 7–10 days.

GYNECOLOGIC PROCEDURES
Potassium Hydroxide (KOH) Prep

- **Indications:** to evaluate vaginal discharge

- **Contraindications:** none

- **What you will need:** vaginal speculum, cotton tip, glass slide, cover slip, 10% KOH solution

- **Procedure:**

  1. During speculum exam, insert a cotton tip into the vagina and collect a sample of vaginal discharge.
  2. Smear specimen on a glass slide.
  3. Add one drop of 10% KOH solution.
  4. Perform the "whiff test" (fishy smell after addition of KOH solution is a sign of bacterial vaginosis).
  5. Place cover slip over the slide, then place slide under the microscope.
  6. Examine the slide at low power (10×) and at higher power (40×) for hyphae, indicating a fungal infection.

Wet Prep

- **Indications:** to evaluate vaginal discharge

- **Contraindications:** none

- **What you will need:** vaginal speculum, cotton tip moistened with sterile water, glass slide, cover slip

- **Procedure:**

  1. During speculum exam, insert moistened cotton tip into vagina and collect a sample of vaginal discharge.
  2. Smear specimen on glass slide; place cover slip over the slide.

3. Examine the slide at low power (10×) and at higher power (40×) if necessary for clue cells (bacterial vaginosis) and motile trichomonads (trichomoniasis).

SURGICAL PROCEDURES
Joint Aspiration/Injection

- **Indications:** Joint effusion, steroid injection, rule out infection.

- **Contraindications:** Infection in skin overlying injection site; steroid injection is contraindicated in infected joints.

- **What you will need:** Betadine, 1–2% lidocaine, 25-gauge needle, 18- or 20-gauge needle, 20-mL syringe, steroid preparation (if injecting joint) in a syringe.

- **Procedure:**

  1. Palpate extensor surface of joint; find and mark spot for aspiration. In the knee, the most common approach is the anteromedial approach, with the needle placed approximately 1 cm below the patella.
  2. Clean the skin with Betadine.
  3. Using the 25-gauge needle, infiltrate the skin with lidocaine for anesthesia.
  4. Gently slide 18- or 20-gauge needle into the joint. You may hear a "pop" as the needle goes into joint.
  5. Aspirate fluid into 20-mL syringe.
  6. If you are also injecting joint, carefully remove 20-mL syringe and attach syringe with the steroid preparation.
  7. Gently inject steroid into joint.
  8. Remove needle and apply pressure to site until hemostasis is achieved.
  9. Send joint fluid for gram stain and culture, glucose, crystals, cytology, cell count, and differential. Place small amount on a slide to examine under polarized light for crystals.

Incision and Drainage

- **Indication:** drainage of a cutaneous abscess

- **Contraindications:** very large abscess (relative contraindication)

- **What you will need:** Betadine, 25-gauge needle and syringe, scalpel (most commonly 10-blade), sterile gauze, sterile water or saline, 1% lidocaine, cotton tip to explore the wound

- **Procedure:**

  1. Palpate area for fluctuance. Clean area with Betadine.
  2. Using the 25-gauge needle, inject skin and make a wheal with 1% lidocaine.
  3. Using scalpel, make incision into center of the abscess.

4. Drain abscess by gently pushing fluid out of incision with sterile gauze pads.
5. If there is any doubt as to the extent of the abscess, use a sterile cotton tip applicator to explore wound.
6. Débride any dead tissue; irrigate if necessary.
7. For large abscesses, extend incision until it is large enough for packing. For small abscesses, allow wound to close via secondary intention.
8. Use wet-to-dry dressing with dressing changes daily until granulation tissue is present. At that point, the wound can be allowed to close, or it may need a skin graft.

Final Touches

What doesn't kill you makes you stronger . . .

- Listen carefully to your patients; communicate with your patients and their families.

- Resident's rule of thumb: number of complaints is inversely proportional to number of diseases.

- Try to focus on one or two complaints per visit—you can always make a follow-up appointment.

- Remember, an ounce of prevention is worth a pound of cure.

- Follow up on all tests.

- Be nice to the support staff—they can make your clinic much more pleasant.

- Use your ancillary services (social workers, dieticians, etc).

- Drug seekers: just say no.

- Think carefully before writing your pager number or Drug Enforcement Agency number on a prescription.

- Paperwork is not the enemy, just a nuisance.

- Caring about your patients is the best thing you can do for them.

Patient Data Tracking Form

Name	Allergies	
Date of Birth	Medication	Reaction
Telephone Number		
Pharmacy/Phone Number		
Height		
Weight		
BMI		

Medical Conditions/Hospitalizations/ Surgeries	Current Medications	

Health Maintenance		Diagnostic Studies	
Complete physical exam			
Tests			
Pap smear			
Clinical breast exam			
Mammogram			
Colon cancer screening			
Prostate cancer screening			
Cholesterol screening			
DEXA scan			
PPD			
Health Guidance		**Immunizations**	
Alcohol screening		Influenza	
Domestic violence screen		Pneumovax	
Exercise		Tetanus	
Seat belts/helmets		Hepatitis A	
Smoking		Hepatitis B	

Index

Note: Page numbers followed by *f* refer to figures; page numbers followed by *t* refer to tables.

Index

Index